Eye Emergencies

Eye Emergencies

Diagnosis and management

Lennox A. Webb FRCS, FRCOphth
Senior Registrar, Tennent Institute of Ophthalmology
Glasgow, UK

With a Foreword by Jack J. Kanski

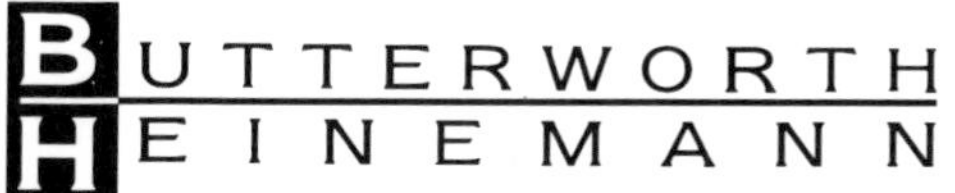

Butterworth-Heinemann Ltd
Linacre House, Jordan Hill, Oxford OX2 8DP

A member of the Reed Elsevier plc group

OXFORD LONDON BOSTON
MUNICH NEW DELHI SINGAPORE SYDNEY
TOKYO TORONTO WELLINGTON

First edition 1995

British Library Cataloguing in Publication Data
A catalogue record for this book is available from the British Library

ISBN 0 7506 2015 3

Library of Congress Cataloguing in Publication Data
A catalogue record for this book is available from the Library of Congress

Phototypeset by Wilmaset Ltd, Wirral
Printed in Great Britain by
The University Press, Cambridge

Contents

Foreword

The casualty officer or general practitioner presented with an eye problem requires a practical pragmatic guide for initial management. This text works on the assumption that the reader has little or no knowledge of the subject, and suggests relevant questions to ask for the majority of common eye problems in a manner designed to ensure that serious pathology is not overlooked. It is not a text which enters into detailed discussion of problems, and is not designed to do so, but simply offers sound guidance to non-ophthalmologists on the management of common eye problems, whether they are true emergencies, or more chronic in nature.

Jack J. Kanski

Preface

There are few true eye emergencies, but a substantial proportion of patients attending the emergency department or general practitioner present with eye problems. These are often a source of despair to the medical officer involved who will often possess only a rudimentary knowledge of ophthalmology. This text assumes the user has little or no experience of the subject and aims to guide the practitioner to the likely diagnosis on the basis of the presenting symptoms or signs. A step-by-step approach is used for both diagnosis and management. The salient features of each condition are given to help identification, and a plan for the disposal of each case is detailed. With the increasing prominence of litigation, pitfalls and how to avoid these have been emphasized where these are most likely to occur. Whereas the majority of eye problems presenting to casualty or the general practitioner are covered in this text, gaps will exist and, where these occur, they should be discussed with the on-call ophthalmologist. Cross-referencing is widely used throughout; however, some topics are deliberately repeated if they fall under two or more headings to allow the user to read through the management of specific problems without having to refer backwards or forwards repeatedly. Finally, it should be remembered that different units will have different management protocols, and that this text is simply a 'core' guide.

Acknowledgements

I am extremely grateful to the following colleagues for taking the time and care to review this manuscript and for making many helpful suggestions:

Mr J. J. Kanski, Consultant Ophthalmologist, Prince Charles Eye Unit, Windsor

Dr S. M. Macleod, Senior House Officer, Tennent Institute of Ophthalmology, Glasgow

Dr C. J. Shadbolt, General Practitioner, Glasgow

My thanks also to Dr T. Patel, Dr H. Ihmaidat, Dr C. O'Neil, Dr R. Metcalfe and Mrs D. Melville for their contributions to this text, and to Ms C. Makepeace and Mr T. Brown at Butterworth-Heinemann for their assistance and support.

Plates 1–14 courtesy of Mr J. J. Kanski

1

Basic examination

Whilst detailed examination technique for each major presenting complaint is described at the beginning of the relevant chapter, a *basic examination* should cover the following:

Lids and orbit

Look for erythema, which may be localized (styes and cysts) or more generalized (orbital cellulitis, Plate 1). Proptosis (protruding eyes) or a staring appearance may indicate dysthyroid eye disease or a mass behind the eye. A drooping eye lid (ptosis) may be associated with a III nerve palsy.

Visual acuity (VA)

Always document this for each eye individually (Fig. 1.2, p. 4). Use correct glasses (i.e. not reading glasses for a 6-metre Snellen visual acuity) or contact lenses if usually worn. Use a pinhole (see below) if the patient has not brought glasses with them.

Normal vision is 6/6 (= 20/20), although for some patients less than this is usual, particularly if there is a history of squint or lazy eye (amblyopia). In the elderly, vision is frequently below this due to cataract or age-related degeneration of the retina.

For example, *6/18*: the 6 indicates the distance, 6 metres, between patient and test chart and the 18 indicates that the text read by the patient is of a size that would be read at 18 metres by a normally sighted

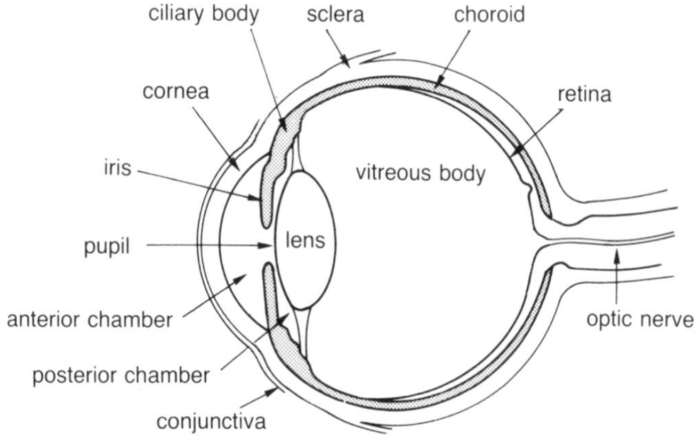

Fig. 1.1.

person, i.e. the patient's vision is subnormal. Figure 1.2, the test chart, uses smaller figures than the full-size Snellen chart and should be held approximately 3 metres from the patient.

A *pinhole* is simply as stated – a small hole or group of holes in a piece of card or plastic, which corrects VA to approximately that achieved with glasses. Make one by pushing a needle through a piece of card or paper, if one is not available.

Eye movements

If defective, and of recent onset, the patient usually complains of double vision. Use a light at least 60 cm from the patient, tell him or her to keep their head still (hold it, if necessary), and ask the patient to follow the light as you move it to eight positions (Fig. 1.3): left, left and up, left and down, right, right and up, right and down, straight up and straight down.

Ask the patient if they see double when looking at the light straight ahead, or in any of the positions tested.

Conjunctiva and sclera

Look for injection, haemorrhage, discharge and swelling (Plates 2 and 3).

Cornea

This should be clear, with a bright, smooth surface. Look for abrasions (Plate 4) and foreign bodies, which may be underneath the upper lid (Plate 5) Evert the upper lid (Fig. 1.4, p. 7) and look for these.

Pupils

These should be round, equal in size and react briskly to a bright light. In the elderly the pupil is often smaller and reacts sluggishly. Look for an afferent pupil defect (APD – see below), which may be present even with normal VA and indicates optic nerve or gross retinal dysfunction. Check the red reflex (see below).

Afferent pupil defect

Shine a bright light for 2 seconds into one pupil, then switch briskly to the other side again for 2 full seconds. Don't do it faster, or you may miss the sign. If one pupil dilates as you shine the light at it, an afferent defect is present.

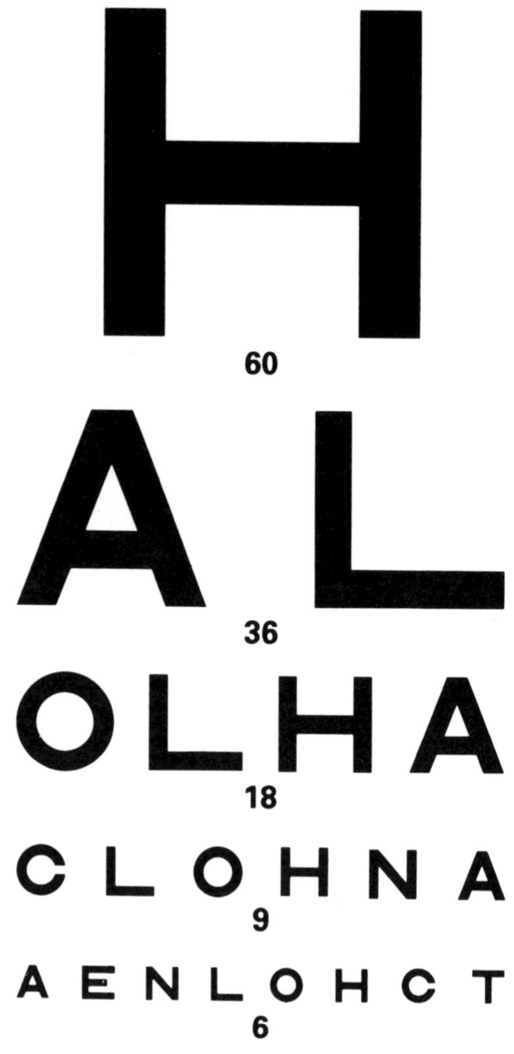

Fig. 1.2. (a) Distance chart – use at 3 metres.

TEST TYPES

N.5.

Now we have reached the trees—the beautiful trees! never so beautiful as to-day. Imagine the effect of a straight and regular double avenue of oaks, nearly a mile long, arching over-head, and closing into perspective like the roof and columns of a cathedral, every tree and branch encrusted with the bright and delicate congelation of hoar-frost, white and pure as snow, delicate and defined as carved ivory. How

— numerous renew assurance our sense ewe camera acorn assess cocoa source essence err —

N.8.

a wide view over four counties—a landscape of snow. A deep lane leads abruptly down the hill; a mere narrow cart-track, sinking between high banks clothed with fern and furze and low broom, crowned with luxuriant

— cam macaroon overseas race ocean excess nurse answer raven —

N.12.

this is rime in its loveliest form ! And there is still a berry here and there on the holly, "blushing in its natural coral," through the delicate tracery,

— same accrue car oxen recover ensnare —

N.18.

wren, "that shadow of a bird," as White, of Selbourne, calls it,

— severe room caravan —

N.36.

amongst the

— occur —

Fig. 1.2. (b) Reading visual acuity charts – use at 30 cm.

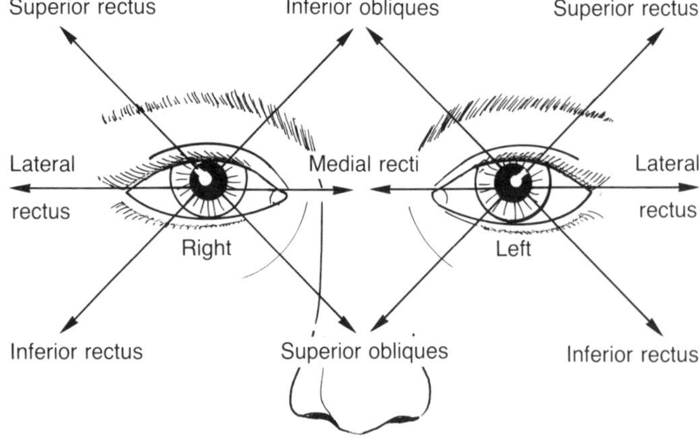

Fig. 1.3. Direction of action of extraocular muscles.

Red reflex

Look through an ophthalmoscope at the pupil from about 45 cm. A red reflex is usually seen from the retina (as in some flash photos, when the subject appears to have red pupils). Opacities such as cataract and vitreous haemorrhage, or surface irregularities such as corneal abrasions, block or reduce this reflex.

Fundus

You should observe three regions using a direct ophthalmoscope:

1. Optic disc – for cupping, pallor, swelling and haemorrhages (Plate 6).
2. Peripheral retina – for detachment.
3. Central retina – for haemorrhages (Plate 7) and pigmentary change.

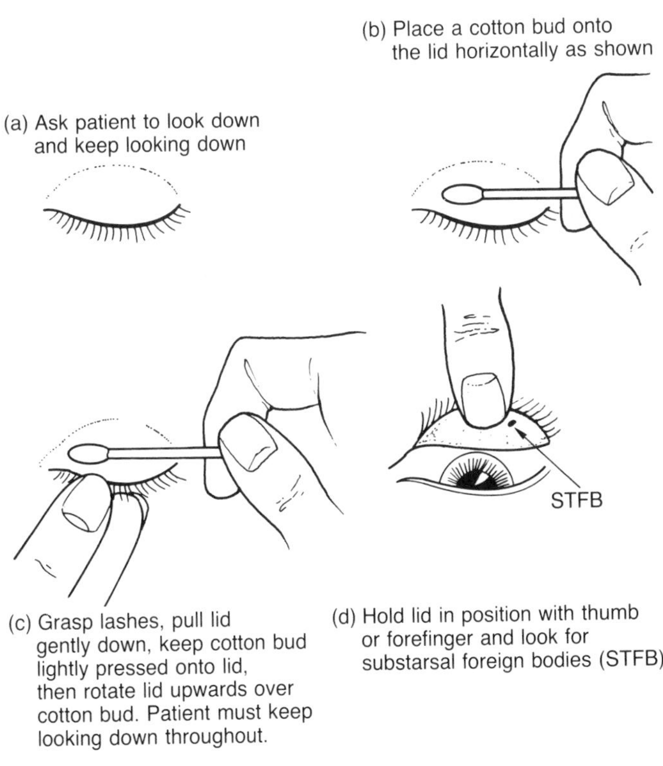

Fig. 1.4. Eversion of upper lid.

No fundal view may be due to a very small pupil, cataract or vitreous haemorrhage. Document the fact if no view is visible.

Visual fields

Common defects are shown in Figure 1.5. A quick screen is all that is required in those with suspected neurological field defects (e.g. strokes).

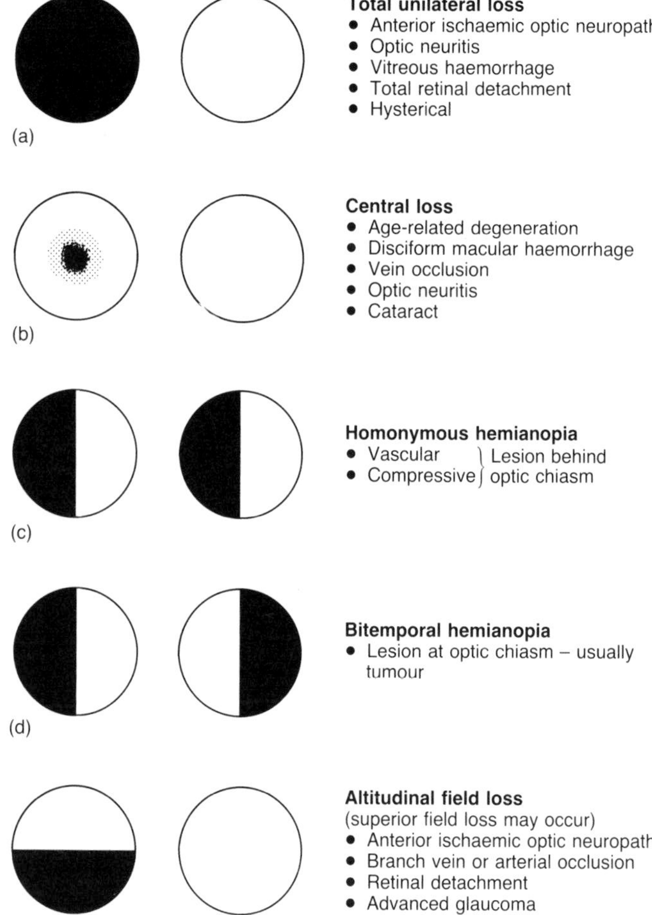

Fig. 1.5. Visual field defects.

1. Sit directly in front of the patient at about 1 metre.
2. Get the patient to cover one eye (without pressing it) and look straight into your eye on the same side (i.e. patient's left eye looking into your right, and vice versa).
3. Ensure that the patient keeps fixing on your eye (very important) and ask if he or she is aware of your hair, nose, mouth, neck, collar – if yes, central vision is grossly intact.
4. Hold an outstretched index finger in each field quadrant, waggle it slightly and ask if the patient sees this movement. Move in centrally until he or she does. Temporally, patients should be able to see an object at least in the same plane as their own eyes. It is not necessary for you also to close an eye and compare their field with yours.

This is a basic visual field test (confrontation field) and will not detect all defects but is sufficient in an emergency room setting.

Pitfalls

Failure to:

1. Carefully document the history, the fact that you have adequately examined the patient, and your clinical findings.
2. Check and document VA in each eye individually.
3. X-ray cases of trauma involving high velocity metal, glass, stone, etc.
4. Refer if there is any suspicion of penetrating injury.

Tips on using the slitlamp

1. Make sure it is plugged in.
2. The patient should have their chin firmly on the chin rest, and their forehead right up against the forehead rest.
3. Adjust the height of the lamp to suit the patient. The Haag–Streit slitlamp has a height adjuster lever just under the front of the table mount.
4. The brightness control is adjacent to the on-off switch. Start on a low setting initially.
5. A silver knurled knob near the top of the machine controls the height of the slit beam and the blue light for looking at the cornea after staining with fluorescein.

2

Red eye

This common complaint is usually due to:

1. Conjunctivitis
2. Corneal foreign body
3. Corneal abrasion
4. Ingrowing eyelashes
5. Subconjunctival haemorrhage
6. Iritis
7. Trauma (p. 116) – chemical injury (p. 38)

Six simple questions will help identify the cause in the majority of cases:

1. Was the patient drilling, welding or grinding?
2. Is there a history of trauma?
3. Is it painful?
4. Is vision reduced?
5. Was the onset acute or chronic?
6. Is there a previous history of eye ulcers?

Which category applies?

1. Acute painful unilateral p. 12
2. Acute painful bilateral p. 34
3. Acute painless unilateral p. 48
4. Acute painless bilateral p. 54
5. Chronic red eye p. 59
6. Trauma (p. 116) – unilateral or bilateral

An accurate history is essential to identify other less common causes prior to examination, and relevant questions are detailed below for each category of complaint.

Red eye – acute onset, painful, unilateral

Common causes

Corneal abrasion p. 16
Corneal foreign body p. 18
Subtarsal foreign body p. 20
Ingrowing lashes p. 21
Iritis p. 23
Contact lens-related pp. 24, 135
Trauma (p. 116) – chemical injury (p. 38)

Less common causes

Corneal ulcer p. 27
Penetrating/blunt injury p. 116
Previous surgery p. 29
Acute glaucoma p. 30
Scleritis/episcleritis p. 31
Shingles p. 33

Relevant questions

1. *Was the patient drilling, grinding, welding or undertaking any other activity with a high risk of corneal foreign body?*
   If a high-velocity particle involved – usually as a result of metal striking metal, always consider a penetrating eye injury (Plate 8). Occurs most frequently in industrial workers, car mechanics, DIY.
2. *Is looking at light painful* (photophobia)*?*

This suggests inflammation within the eye such as iritis. This may be secondary to other trauma, e.g. blunt injury or severe abrasion.

3. *Is there any history of trauma to the eye – past or present?*
   Corneal abrasions (Plate 4) are frequently caused by an infant's fingernail, newspapers and foreign bodies. A previous abrasion may recurrently break down, usually on awakening from sleep (recurrent erosion).
4. *Does the patient wear contact lenses?*
   Overworn or poorly cleaned contact lenses may induce corneal abrasions or ulcers.
5. *Has the patient had an eye operation recently or in the past?*
   Irritation due to sutures is not uncommon following cataract and squint surgery (see Fig. 10.1, p. 168).

   Pain following retinal detachment surgery is common for several days postoperatively.
6. *Has the patient had iritis (eye inflammation) in the past?*
   Young men with ankylosing spondylitis often have recurrent iritis.
7. *Is vision blurred?*
   This occurs in most cases of painful red eye, often due to excess watering, or a central corneal abrasion. Acute glaucoma causes corneal clouding and occurs predominantly in the elderly.

Eye examination

External

The patient may be unable to open the eye due to pain and photophobia.

If due to surface trauma, such as a corneal abrasion or foreign body, instil a drop of topical anaesthetic (benoxinate 0.4% or amethocaine 1.0%). This may allow you to continue the examination.

Lids

Examine for lacerations or site of entry of high-velocity particles (see Fig. 5.2, p. 128). Evert the upper lid and look for subtarsal foreign bodies, unless a penetrating injury is obvious, in which case this procedure should not be undertaken. Look for ingrowing eyelashes. To evert the upper lid (see Fig. 1.4, p. 7).

Orbit

Feel the orbital rim for tenderness or rim fractures.

Visual acuity (VA)

May be markedly reduced following a central corneal abrasion, contact lens overwear and acute glaucoma but is usually normal or only minimally reduced with corneal foreign bodies, iritis or episcleritis. A penetrating injury may lead to gross or minimal visual loss depending upon the degree of intraocular damage.

Pupil

Pupil constriction often occurs in iritis and corneal abrasions. A fixed, oval pupil in the presence of a hazy cornea in an elderly patient indicates acute glaucoma. A distorted pupil with a history of trauma may signify a penetrating injury.

Conjunctiva

Conjunctival haemorrhage (Plate 3) or chemosis (oedematous swelling) may mask an underlying scleral wound. Localized inflammation suggests episcleritis. Circumferential conjunctival injection near the cornea in the presence of photophobia suggests uveitis (Plate 2). Examine the conjunctival fornices (under the lids) for foreign bodies, including contact lenses. Evert the upper lid (Fig. 1.4, p. 7).

Cornea

Stain the cornea with dilute fluorescein and look for corneal staining suggestive of an abrasion (Plate 4) or corneal ulcer (Plate 9). Look for corneal foreign bodies, particularly if the history is suggestive. Examine under the upper eyelid, provided there is no suggestion of a penetrating injury. Foreign bodies frequently lodge at this site and cause characteristic abrasions on the upper cornea (Plate 5).

A distorted pupil may indicate a penetrating injury of the cornea or sclera. To examine for leaking aqueous, instil 2% fluorescein and observe under a blue light. Absence of a leak does not imply absence of a penetrating injury, as the wound may self-seal.

A cloudy cornea in an elderly patient associated with pain, debility and reduced vision suggests acute glaucoma (p. 30).

Anterior chamber

Look for:

1. A hyphaema (blood level) in trauma (Plate 11).
2. A hypopyon (white level of inflammatory or pus cells, Plate 9) associated with intraocular infection (endophthalmitis) or severe uveitis.

Lens

A cataract may be associated with a penetrating injury.

Corneal abrasion

Features

This is usually caused by a foreign body, child's fingernail, mascara brushes, twigs and plants. The eye is acutely painful and waters profusely. Abraded cornea appears green under a blue light when stained with fluorescein (Plates 4 and 5).

Management

1. Instil a drop of local anaesthetic to allow examination.

2. Instil a drop of fluorescein. Abraded cornea appears green under a blue light, but is usually visible even under a white light.

3. Ensure there is no corneal foreign body. Linear corneal abrasions (Plate 5) in the upper part of the cornea are characteristic of a subtarsal foreign body. The upper lid should be everted in all abrasions to ensure that this is not missed.

To evert the upper lid, ask the patient to look down, and keep looking down (see Fig. 1.4, p. 7). Place the wooden stick of a cotton bud horizontally across the mid-portion of the upper lid, grasp the eyelashes firmly and gently rotate the lid upwards over the stick.

4. Remove any foreign bodies by firmly wiping with a cotton bud.

5. Instil a drop of homatropine 1% or cyclopentolate 1% (mydrilate) to dilate the pupil and reduce pain secondary to iris spasm.
6. Instil chloramphenicol ointment 1% stat.
7. Patch the eye with two eye pads:
   (a) Fold one patch in half and place over the closed eye.
   (b) Place the other patch on top and tape down firmly.
8. Leave patches on for 24 hours. Although patching may not speed healing and are not essential, patients often prefer them.
9. Chloramphenicol ointment 1% b.d. for 3 days.

To instil ointment

Pull down the lower lid and squeeze a short line of ointment into the gutter formed between the inner surface of the lower lid and the eye. Most comes out on blinking, but sufficient is usually retained for therapeutic effect.

Advise the patient that the eye will become painful again once the local anaesthetic has worn off – usually within half an hour. Simple analgesia, e.g. paracetamol 1g 6-hourly, is all that is required, and may help reduce symptoms. Complete healing of the abrasion usually takes up to 48 hours.

Infants

Infants may need to be wrapped in a blanket to restrain limbs and allow examination.

Do not patch.

Always discuss with an ophthalmologist.

Referral

Referral is not required unless there is failure to heal within 48 hours, in which case refer to the ophthalmologist within a further 24 hours.

Follow-up

This is only required if the abrasion is very large, or bilateral. The patient should be reviewed the following day.

Pitfalls

Failure to examine subtarsally for a foreign body.

Corneal foreign body

Features

Metallic corneal foreign bodies are common and usually occur when drilling, grinding or welding. Dried-paint foreign bodies may be found in painters and decorators and organic foreign bodies in gardeners. Pain may be minimal or acute. Profuse watering is common.

Management

1. Instil a drop of topical anaesthetic.
2. Dislodge the foreign body with an orange needle.
   (a) Mount the needle on a 2 ml syringe, which acts as a handle and gives you greater control.
   (b) Tell the patient what you are about to do, and

reassure him or her that the needle does not go into the eye.

(c) Hold the patient's upper lid to prevent blinking as follows:
   (i) Ask the patient to look down.
   (ii) Place your thumb on the lower border of the upper lid and elevate the lid.
   (iii) Ask the patient to look straight ahead.

(d) Gently try to remove the foreign body with the tip of the needle at a glancing (shallow) angle to the corneal surface (corneal thickness is only 0.5 mm).

(e) Once the foreign body is dislodged, pick it up with a cotton bud, as this is easier than attempting to remove it from the surface of a watering eye with the needle.

3. If a rust-ring remains around the foreign body site after removal, attempt to remove this as well. If it proves difficult, leave it for the ophthalmologist. It is often easier to remove after 24–48 hours.

4. Instil a drop of cyclopentolate 1% (Mydrilate) if the eye is very inflamed (if not, omit this).

5. Instil chloramphenicol ointment 1%.

6. Pad the eye with two eye pads for 24 hours:
   (a) Fold one patch in half and place over the closed eye.
   (b) Place the other patch on top and tape down firmly.

7. Advise patient that the eye will be painful once the topical anaesthetic has worn off – usually within half an hour – but should settle within 24 hours.

Referral

Refer to the ophthalmologist within 24 hours if you are unable to remove the foreign body completely.

Follow-up

Follow-up is not required.

Pitfalls

Failure to:

- Suspect a penetrating injury.
- Examine the other eye for a foreign body.
- Look for subtarsal foreign bodies (STFB).

Subtarsal foreign body (STFB)

Features

Suspect an STFB if linear abrasions are seen in the upper cornea (Plate 5) associated with pain or low-grade irritation.

Associations

Frequently following debris blown into eye by wind. Always suspect these in children presenting with a red eye.

Management

1. Instil a drop of topical anaesthetic.
2. Evert the upper lid over a cotton bud (see Fig. 1.4, p. 7).
3. Remove the foreign body with a firm wipe from a cotton bud.
4. Instil a drop of homatropine 1% or cyclopentolate 1% (Mydrilate) if patient is photophobic.

5. Instil chloramphenicol ointment 1%.
6. Pad with two eye pads for 24 hours if multiple abrasions are present:
   (a) Fold one patch in half and place over the closed eye.
   (b) Place the other patch on top and tape down firmly.
7. Advise the patient that the eye will be painful once the topical anaesthetic has worn off – usually in half an hour – but should settle within 24 hours.

Referral and follow-up

Not required unless fails to settle within 48 hours, in which case refer to the ophthalmologist within a further 24 hours.

Pitfalls

Failure to:

- Suspect a penetrating injury.
- Examine other eye for foreign body.

Ingrowing lashes (trichiasis)

Features

This is common and recurrent, usually in the elderly.

Management

1. Ensure that the lid has not turned in on itself such that the lashes are in contact with the globe

(entropion, Fig. 2.1a). This is common in the elderly.

2. If no entropion is present, epilate (pull out) the offending lashes with forceps.
3. If entropion is present, use steristrips to pull the lower lid off the globe (Fig. 2.1b), as follows:
   (a) Dry the skin.
   (b) Place one end of a steristrip on the skin just below the lashes.

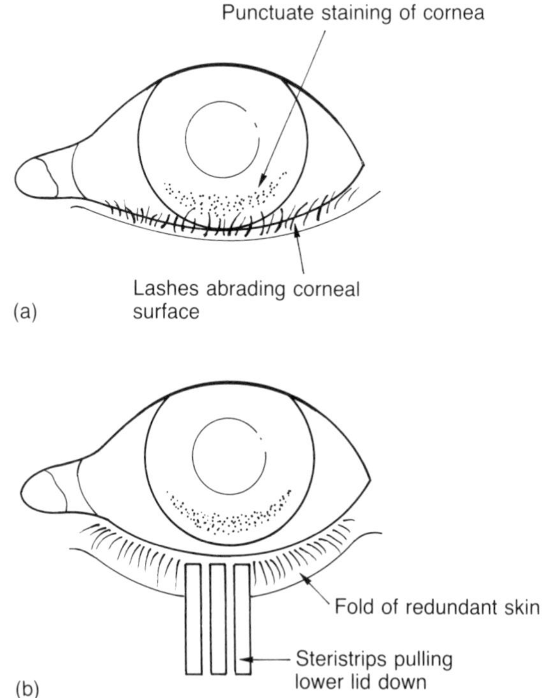

Fig. 2.1. (a) Entropion. (b) Temporary correction using steristrips.

(c) Pull down gently until lashes are pulled off the globe.
(d) Stick other end on to cheek.
(e) Use three steristrips in a row.

4. Chloramphenicol ointment 1% b.d. for 5 days.

Referral

If entropion is present, refer to ophthalmology outpatient department (soon – 48 hours). If there is no entropion, but the problem is recurrent, organize a routine outpatient appointment, otherwise discharge.

Follow-up

On an as-required basis only, not routinely.

Iritis (uveitis)

Features

Photophobia (light is painful), perilimbal (junction between the cornea and sclera) or diffuse injection (plate 2), a small pupil and ocular tenderness. The history often indicates previous episodes, particularly in men with ankylosing spondylitis.

Management

1. Listen to patients if they state that this is a recurrent problem – they are usually well-versed in the appropriate management.

2. Ensure that the patient does not have a dendritic ulcer (Plate 10), by staining the cornea with fluorescein.
3. If the iritis is mild and the patient is not distressed, treat as follows:
   (a) Dexamethasone 0.1% (Maxidex) drops 2 hourly. *Only start steroids if you are confident of the diagnosis.*
   (b) Cyclopentolate 1% (Mydrilate) drops t.i.d. Check that the pupil dilates with this. If it is adherent to the lens (posterior synechiae), a stronger dilating agent, e.g. Atropine 1% is required.

Referral

Mild cases should be seen by the ophthalmologist within 24 hours. Severe cases should be discussed immediately.

Follow-up

Ophthalmologist only.

Pitfalls

Iritis is often mistreated as conjunctivitis. Photophobia and pain are common to iritis, and rare in conjunctivitis.

Contact lens overwear

Features

This is common and usually occurs as a result of

failure to remove contact lenses before sleeping. Pain and profuse watering occur.

Management

1. Confirm that contact lenses have been removed.
2. Instil a drop of topical anaesthetic if the patient is unable to open the eyes.
3. Stain the cornea with fluorescein and observe under a blue light. A diffuse central pattern of staining is common, often in both eyes.
4. Ensure there is no corneal ulcer (p. 27).
5. Instil chloramphenicol ointment 1%.
6. Instil a drop of homatropine 1% or cyclopentolate 1% (Mydrilate).
7. Patch the eye, or the worst eye if both eyes are involved, with two patches for 24 hours:
   (a) Fold one patch in half and place over the closed eye.
   (b) Place the other patch on top and tape down firmly.
8. Advise the patient to leave out contact lenses during treatment.

Referral and follow-up

Not required unless an ulcer is present (p. 27).

Lost contact lens

Features

This may occur spontaneously or following trauma, typically sports-related. Pain may be absent.

Management

1. Ensure that the patient has not in fact removed the lens.
2. Instil a drop of topical anaesthetic.
3. Examine with a slitlamp if available. Look in the lower conjunctival fornix by making the patient look up whilst you pull the lower lid down. Ask the patient to look left and right whilst looking up, and look for the lens in the folds of conjunctiva.
4. Evert the upper lid as in Figure 1.4, p. 7. Make the patient look left and right again. Place a cotton bud under the upper lid into the upper conjunctival fornix and sweep it once (uncomfortable).
5. If the lens is still not found, instil fluorescein and observe under a blue light. Repeat steps 3 and 4. If the patient has soft lenses, advise before instilling the drop that this will stain the lens. Fluorescein assists in highlighting the lens.
6. If the lens is found, ensure that it is intact. If part is missing, search for this.
7. Discharge on chloramphenicol ointment 1% q.d.s. for 1 week, and advise patient not to reinsert the lens for this period.
8. Patch the eye for 24 hours if abrasions are present.

Referral

Only required if lens is not found, or part is missing. Refer to the ophthalmologist within 24 hours after instilling chloramphenicol ointment, and gently patching the eye.

Follow up

Not required unless severe abrasions are present, in which case review after 24 hours.

Corneal ulcer

Features

This usually occurs in the following cases:

1. Soft contact lens wearers
2. Blepharitis (p. 56) – marginal ulcers
3. Dry eyes
4. Those with a previous history of ulcers or cold sores around the lips (dendritic ulcers).

Contact lens-related ulcers usually have an oval-shaped epithelial defect overlying a white central or peripheral corneal opacity (Plate 9).
Dendritic ulcers (herpes simplex virus, as with cold sores) have a characteristic branching shape and may be multiple (Plate 10).
Ulcers associated with eyelid disease – particularly in those with blepharitis or rosacea (ruddy cheeks and nose) – are often crescent-shaped and at the corneal periphery (marginal ulcers).

Management

1. Instil a drop of fluorescein, ask the patient to blink a few times and observe under a blue light.
   (a) *Contact lens-related ulcers – do not start on antibiotics but discuss with ophthalmologist immediately.*

(b) *Dendritic ulcers*
   (i) Acyclovir 3% (Zovirax) ointment five times a day for 7 days.
   (ii) Cyclopentolate 1% (Mydrilate) drops b.d. if the eye is painful and photophobic (pain with light).
   A small dendritic ulcer will usually resolve within 7–10 days on adequate treatment.

(c) *Marginal ulcers* – Refer as below. Topical steroids are usually required.

Referral

Contact lens-related – immediately to the ophthalmologist.
Dendritic ulcer – ophthalmologist within 24–48 hours if the ulcer is large or has not healed after a week of adequate therapy.
Marginal ulcer – ophthalmologist within 24 hours.
Other ulcer – discuss with ophthalmologist immediately.

Follow-up

Contact lens-related – ophthalmologist only.
Dendritic ulcers – see in 1 week. If healed, discharge, otherwise refer as above. The treatment may then be stopped, and the patient warned to reattend should any symptoms recur.
Marginal and other ulcers – ophthalmologist only.

Pitfall

Never start topical steroids without first discussing with the ophthalmologist.

Previous surgery

This is described in detail in Chapter 10 (p. 167).

Features

Postoperative problems usually involve irritable sutures following cataract or squint surgery (see Fig. 10.1, p. 168), external infection or intraocular infection (endophthalmitis). Pain is common following retinal detachment surgery. Consider rejection in a corneal graft.

Management

Pain or acute reduction in vision must be discussed with the ophthalmologist.

1. Check visual acuity (p. 1) and red reflex (p. 6), as these are profoundly reduced in endophthalmitis.
2. Stain with fluorescein and look for prominent sutures under a blue light. These will be in the upper corneoscleral junction in postoperative cataracts, and in the medial and temporal conjunctiva following squint surgery (Fig. 10.1, p. 168). Corneal staining may be present in graft rejection.
3. Do not attempt to remove any sutures. Give chloramphenicol ointment 1% q.i.d. and refer as below.
4. Examine the anterior chamber for a hypopyon (pus level seen inside the eye, Plate 9), suggesting severe uveitis or endophthalmitis.
5. Examine the conjunctival fornices (gutter between the eye and the lower lid, and the same area for the

upper lid) for protruding explant material used in retinal detachment surgery (white cylinders of sponge).

Referral

With the exception of prominent sutures, which should be treated as above and referred to the ophthalmologist within 24 hours, all other postoperative problems should be discussed with the ophthalmologist immediately. Endophthalmitis requires immediate admission and intensive treatment.

Follow-up

Ophthalmologist only.

Pitfall

Failure to recognize that decreased vision, pain and an absent red reflex indicates endophthalmitis or graft rejection.

Penetrating and blunt injury

This is discussed in the section on trauma (p. 116).

Acute glaucoma

Features

This occurs predominantly in elderly patients, who may be very debilitated as a result of the intense ocular pain. Abdominal pain and vomiting may predominate. The cornea is cloudy, the pupil fixed and semidilated and vision markedly reduced. The eye feels rock hard when palpated through the eyelid.

Management

1. Diamox 500 mg i.v. to reduce intraocular pressure and ocular pain.
2. Pilocarpine 2% drops to both eyes and then every half an hour to the affected eye.
3. Analgesia is very important and often forgotten. Use pethidine 50 mg i.m. stat. This may be adjusted according to the weight of the patient.
4. Antiemetic. Don't give this orally. Prochlorperazine (Stemetil) 12.5 mg i.m or metoclopramide (Maxolon) 10 mg i.m./i.v.

Referral

Admit immediately under the ophthalmologists.

Follow-up

Ophthalmologist only.

Episcleritis

Features

Episcleritis is either asympomatic or mildly irritable. The eye may be diffusely red or, more frequently, only a sector of 'conjunctiva' is involved, usually medially or temporally. An injected tender nodule may be present – nodular episcleritis. Visual acuity is normal.

Management

1. Stain with fluorescein to ensure that the erythema is not secondary to an abrasion (Plates 4 and 5) on the conjunctiva, an ulcer or a foreign body. If staining is present, evert the lids and look for a subtarsal foreign body (p. 20). Ensure there are no aberrant lashes growing inwards, and that there is not a lash in the lacrimal punctum.
2. If asymptomatic, do not treat at all, and reassure the patient that this often clears spontaneously.
3. If symptomatic, start on a non-steroidal anti-inflammatory agent, e.g. flurbiprofen (Froben) 50–100 mg b.d. orally, provided there are no gastrointestinal (GI) contraindications. Warn patient to stop if GI symptoms occur.
4. Do not start on topical steroids.

Referral

Only required if recurrent, or patient is symptomatic. Routine ophthalmology outpatient appointment.

Follow-up

If asymptomatic, no follow-up is required. If treatment as above has been initiated, see in 3–4 days and check that no GI side-effects have occurred. Discharge and stop all treatment after 10 days.

Shingles

Features

Shingles affecting the ophthalmic division of the trigeminal nerve (herpes zoster ophthalmicus, HZO) accounts for 10% of shingles. Eye complications include corneal ulcers, iritis, raised intraocular pressure and periorbital skin vesicles with crusting and subsequent scarring (p. 156).

Management

1. Document visual acuity in each eye. Use a pinhole if required (p. 1).
2. Instil a drop of dilute fluorescein and look for corneal staining.
3. Treat with cyclopentolate 1% (Mydrilate) t.i.d. if the eye is red.
4. If only the eyelids are red or swollen, but the eye itself is white, eye drops are not required. (See p. 156).
5. Acyclovir 3% (Zovirax) ointment is not required.
6. Acyclovir (Zovirax) shingles pack (800 mg 5× day for 1 week p.o.). This can be effective even if several days have elapsed since onset.
7. Analgesia, oral or intramuscular. The pain can be excruciating. Amitriptyline is sometimes effective.

Referral

Ophthalmologist within 24 hours.

Follow-up

Ophthalmologist will follow up if any ocular complications are present, otherwise review (GP) for supportive care.

Red eye – acute, painful, bilateral

There are only a few common causes of acute bilateral painful red eye, most of which relate to trauma or infection.

Chemical injury p. 38.
Welding/grinding p. 39.
Contact lens wear p. 41.
Allergic reaction p. 42.
Bacterial conjunctivitis p. 44.
Viral conjunctivitis p. 45.
Thyroid-related p. 47.

Relevant questions

1. *Was a chemical of any nature splashed into the eye?*
   Wash out with copious amounts of water or saline immediately, before proceeding with further questions or examination (p. 38).
2. *Is there a history of welding or grinding?*
   Welders' flash from ultraviolet light occurs if goggles are not worn. Grinding may lead to bilateral corneal foreign bodies.
3. *Does he or she wear contact lenses?*
   Overwear of contact lenses (usually due to sleep-

ing with lenses in), and failure to rinse them adequately after using cleaning solution is common.

4. *Is there a discharge?*
   Conjunctivitis is rarely painful, but may be irritable and described by the patient as being painful.
5. *Does he or she have sore, irritable eyelid margins?*
   Blepharitis (p. 146) is common and often presents as sore, red, irritable eyes. There is usually a long history of ocular and lid irritation prior to the acute episode, and may be associated with corneal ulcers.
6. *Does he or she use eye drops?*
   Allergies to antibiotic drops are not uncommon. There may be associated lid oedema and erythema.
7. *Has the patient recently had flu or a cold?*
   Viral keratoconjunctivitis may follow upper respiratory tract viral infection.
8. *Is there a history of thyroid disease?*
   Dysthyroid eye disease may present with mild or gross conjunctival chemosis, erythema and discomfort. The patient may be euthyroid, despite ocular involvement.
9. *Is there a history of head injury?*
   A caroticocavernous fistula following trauma is an extremely rare cause of bilateral red eyes. It may occur spontaneously in elderly hypertensives.

Eye examination

External

Look for signs of trauma, particularly chemical injury. Proptosis (bulging appearance to eye) and lid retraction (staring expression) may be present in dysthyroid eye disease.

Visual acuity

This is reduced in most painful eyes due to watering and blepharospasm (eyes squeezed shut), quite apart from other pathology. Instil a drop of topical anaesthetic if blepharospasm is present, as this will relieve discomfort due to corneal surface trauma and will allow further examination. Conjunctivitis rarely leads to reduced vision. Dysthyroid eye disease may lead to loss of vision from corneal exposure or optic nerve compression.

Fields

It is unnecessary to check visual fields (p. 8) unless you suspect compression of the optic nerve. A check of colour vision is useful. Compare the patient's perception of a bright red-coloured object in each eye individually. Loss of red appreciation indicates optic nerve dysfunction.

Pupils

Pupils may be slightly miosed (small) in severe inflammation secondary to any ocular surface disorder, but still react equally to light. An afferent pupil defect (p. 3) may be present in dysthyroid eye disease, indicating optic nerve compression.

Lids

Crusting and erythema around the eyelashes indicates blepharitis. Look for corneal ulcers in association with this condition (p. 27).

Conjunctiva

Injection may be secondary to corneal or intraocular pathology rather than simply conjunctivitis. Instil fluorescein and look for abrasions on the conjunctiva as well as the cornea. Chemical injury may lead to diffuse staining if mild, or gross loss of conjunctival and corneal epithelium. Markedly swollen conjunctiva may be secondary to dysthyroid eye disease.

Cornea

Examine for surface and subtarsal foreign bodies. (pp. 18–20) Stain with fluorescein and look for epithelial defects. Diffuse staining occurs in mild chemical (often contact lens cleaning solution) and ultraviolet light (welding flash) injuries. Gross epithelial loss may occur in chemical injury. Punctate staining may indicate viral keratoconjunctivitis. Simultaneous bilateral dendritic ulcers are extremely rare.

Anterior chamber

Look for signs of inflammation, particularly perilimbal injection. Bilateral acute (painful) uveitis is uncommon, as is bilateral simultaneous acute glaucoma.

Fundus

Engorgement of blood vessels occurs in caroticocavernous fistula.

General examination

Look for other sites of injury in chemical or other trauma and treat appropriately. Examine for signs of hyperthyroidism.

Pitfalls

Bilateral conjunctival chemosis in dysthyroid eye disease may be attributed to an allergy or conjunctivitis.

Chemical injury

Features

Alkali injuries (ammonia, cement, caustic soda, bleach) can rapidly penetrate the cornea and destroy the eye. If the conjunctiva immediately adjacent to the cornea is white, this may indicate destruction of limbal vessels and severe injury. Acid injuries, although potentially severe, do not tend to cause as much intraocular destruction.

Management

1. *Seconds count.* Wash out immediately, before taking a detailed history and examination. Lie the patient on a couch and irrigate the eyes with copious quantities of water or saline. Ensure that the conjunctival fornices (the folds of conjunctiva in the lower lid and underneath the upper lid) are also adequately irrigated, and that no solid particles of chemical are left *in situ*. At least 1 litre per eye should be used – more for alkaline injuries. A 1-litre bag of saline with a drip set on maximum flow provides good irrigation – however, simply use the quickest means available, e.g. head under a tap.
2. Check the pH with litmus paper and stop irrigating only when neutral.

3. Instil topical anaesthetic to allow eye examination.
4. If mild irritant is involved (soaps, hairspray, etc.), examine the cornea after irrigation. Stain with dilute fluorescein and observe under a blue light. If there is minimal epithelial damage, treat as an abrasion (p. 16).

Referral

Acid and alkali injuries must be referred immediately to the ophthalmologist whilst irrigation continues. Mild chemical irritant injuries require no referral.

Follow-up

Not required in cases involving minor irritants. All other cases will be followed up by the ophthalmologist.

Pitfalls

Inadequate irrigation and failure to remove solid debris (particularly concrete) from under the upper lid and lower conjunctival fornix.

A severely injured eye may appear misleadingly white due to destruction of blood vessels.

Injury related to welding and grinding – foreign bodies and flash burns

Features

Acute pain and copious watering are common. A rust-ring may be present in ferrous foreign bodies after just a few hours. Foreign bodies due to simple welding or grinding are superficial and do not penetrate the globe.

Management

1. Instil topical anaesthetic drops to alleviate blepharospasm and allow examination.
2. Instil fluorescein and look under a blue light for abrasions and foreign bodies.
3. Remove foreign bodies if present (p. 18), and then treat as an abrasion (p. 16).
4. Check for subtarsal foreign bodies (p. 20).
5. Instil a drop of homatropine 1% or cyclopentolate 1% (Mydrilate) to both eyes.
6. Instil chloramphenicol ointment 1% into both eyes.
7. Patch the worst eye for 24 hours.

Referral

This is unnecessary unless difficulty is experienced removing a foreign body or rust ring. In this case, treat as above and refer to the ophthalmologist within 24 hours.

Follow-up

Not required.

Pitfall

Do not fail to take an X-ray of the orbit if the history includes hammering or chiselling. Look for evidence of a penetrating injury (Plate 8) or intraocular foreign body (Plate 12).

Contact lens wear-related

Features

Bilateral red eyes following contact lens wear are usually related to overwear, (usually as a result of sleeping with lenses in) failure to rinse adequately after chemically cleaning or acute exacerbation of allergic response to soft lenses. Copious watering and blepharospasm (unable to open eyes) are common.

Management

1. Ensure contact lenses have been removed. If unable to open eyes, proceed to (2) first.
2. Instil a drop of topical anaesthetic to allow examination.
3. Do not instil fluorescein if soft lenses are *in situ*.
4. Once lenses have been removed, stain with fluorescein, and look for abrasions, ulcers or, more commonly, diffuse punctate staining which indicates overwear or chemical injury due to cleaning solution.
5. Irrigate if history implicates contact lens cleaning solution.
6. In severe cases, instil a drop of homatropine 1% or cyclopentolate 1% (Mydrilate) to relieve ciliary muscle spasm and pain.
7. Instil chloramphenicol ointment 1% into each eye.

8. Treat diffuse staining as an abrasion (p. 16) and patch the worst eye.
9. If an ulcer is present (p. 27) refer as below.
10. Instruct patient to leave out contact lenses until they have been checked for foreign bodies by his or her optician, and not to reinsert them for a minimum of 1 week.

Referral

Discuss with the ophthalmologist if a corneal ulcer is present (p. 27).

Severe bilateral punctate staining secondary to overwear or cleaning solution should be reviewed within 24 hours and, if not improving, discussed with the ophthalmologist.

Advise the patient to attend optician, as in (10) above.

Follow-up

Not required. Leave to the ophthalmologist if involved.

Allergic reaction to eye drops or contact lenses

Features

Allergies typically occur to antibiotic eye drops started for conjunctivitis. In conjunction with red eyes, the periorbital skin may be erythematous, with lower-lid and upper-cheek oedema.

Management

1. Identify any new drops recently started – usually for conjunctivitis.
2. Remove contact lenses if *in situ*. Instil topical anaesthetic to relieve discomfort and assist examination.
3. Stop any new antibiotic drops, and if required replace with an alternative. Most common antibiotic drops used are chloramphenicol, Genticin and Fucithalmic.
4. Glaucoma drops should not be stopped before discussing with the ophthalmologist. The most commonly used glaucoma drops, e.g. Timoptol, pilocarpine, Betagan and Betoptic rarely cause red eyes. Atropine (used in rubeotic glaucoma) and Propine are most frequently associated with allergic reactions.
5. Cold compresses over both eyes improve comfort and reduce swelling.
6. Contact lenses should not be replaced until reviewed by ophthalmologist.

Referral

All cases should be seen by the ophthalmologist within 24 hours to modify treatment if required.

Follow-up

Ophthalmologist will arrange this if required.

Conjunctivitis

Features

Conjunctivitis (Plate 2) rarely leads to a painful eye unless the cornea is also involved, as in viral kerato-conjunctivitis. Patients may complain of pain, which on questioning is simply irritation. A discharge indicates bacterial conjunctivitis (p. 50), whereas excess lacrimation (watering) is associated with viral infections (p. 45).

Management

1. Stain the cornea with fluorescein and look for characteristic punctate staining of adenovirus (p. 46).
2. Follicles – pale grey/pink gelatinous-looking globules within the conjunctiva – indicate viral disease. If associated with a discharge in sexually active individuals, consider *Chlamydia* and take swabs.
3. Treat with chloramphenicol drops 0.5% q.d.s. to both eyes for 10 days. If *Chlamydia* is suspected, treat with tetracycline ointment 1% q.d.s. for 3 weeks, in addition to oral tetracycline 250 mg p.o. q.d.s. for 3 weeks. Sexual partners also require treatment.
4. If patient has already been treated with no effect (first-line therapy is usually chloramphenicol) take a conjunctival swab, by asking the patient to look up and sweeping the lower conjunctival fornix with the swab.
5. Treat with an alternative antibiotic in the case of

bacterial conjunctivitis, such as gentamicin ointment 0.3% (Genticin) q.d.s. or fusidic acid 1% (Fucithalmic) ointment b.d.

Referral

This is not required unless symptoms do not improve or worsen over 3–4 days. If visual loss or severe pain is present, discuss with the ophthalmologist and refer within 24 hours. *Infants* – discuss with ophthalmologist immediately. *Chlamydia* may lead to severe local and systemic complications.

Follow-up

Not required, other than by ophthalmologists, as above.

Viral keratoconjunctivitis

Features

This is usually an adenoviral infection which occurs after an upper airway respiratory tract infection, or contact with similarly affected individuals. Adenovirus has a naturally resolving course but corneal involvement, if present, may last for months. Bilateral dendritic ulceration is rare but should be considered if there has been a previous history of these, cold sores or immunosuppression.

Management

1. Instil a drop of topical anaesthetic if the patient is unable to open their eyes.
2. Stain the cornea with fluorescein.
3. Adenovirus stains lightly as multiple punctate spots, best seen under the slitlamp, whereas dendritic ulcers have a characteristic branching pattern (Plate 10).
4. If you suspect adenovirus, discharge on chloramphenicol drops q.d.s. to each eye for 3 weeks.
5. If bilateral dendritic ulcers are present, treat with acyclovir 3% (Zovirax) ointment five times daily (p. 28) and take a differential full blood count (consider immunosuppression).

Wash your hands thoroughly – adenovirus is extremely contagious and easily spreads to healthcare workers.

Referral

Adenovirus – no referral required unless symptoms fail to improve over 2 weeks.

Bilateral dendritic ulcers are rare and should be reviewed by the ophthalmologist within 24 hours. Admit under physicians if immunosuppression is suspected, as i.v. acyclovir may be required.

Follow-up

Not required, other than by ophthalmologist, as above.

Dysthyroid eye disease

Features

This may occur in a euthyroid patient. The eyes may be minimally or grossly injected, and have a staring appearance. Sight-threatening complications may occur as a result of corneal exposure secondary to proptosis and optic nerve compression secondary to increased orbital pressure. Gross chemosis (swelling and oedema of the conjunctiva) may be present. Diplopia is common.

Management

1. Document visual acuity in each eye with glasses or pinhole if required (p. 1).
2. An afferent pupil defect (p. 3) indicates compression of the optic nerve and must be referred immediately.
3. Stain the cornea with fluorescein and look for staining. If present, this indicates corneal exposure. Treat with Lacri-Lube ointment t.d.s.

Referral

Reduction in vision or pupil defect – immediately to ophthalmologist.
Corneal staining – ophthalmologist within 24 hours after treatment as above.
Cases with no sign of corneal exposure or optic nerve dysfunction – ophthalmologist within 48 hours.

Follow-up

Ophthalmologist only, who will arrange further referral as required.

Pitfall

Dysthyroid conjunctival chemosis may be treated inappropriately as conjunctivitis. There is no discharge in dysthyroid eye disease.

Red eye – acute, painless unilateral

Main causes

1. Conjunctivitis (p. 50)
2. Subconjunctival haemorrhage (p. 51)
3. Episcleritis (p. 52)
4. Allergic reaction (pp. 42, 57)

Relevant questions

1. *Is there any discharge?*
   Bacterial conjunctivitis is often associated with a yellow or white discharge. A watery discharge may occur in a viral or an incompletely treated bacterial conjunctivitis (Plate 2).
2. *Is there a history of any Valsalva manoeuvre or trauma – for instance, carrying heavy weights, coughing or sneezing fits?*
   Subconjunctival haemorrhage may occur following the above as a result of a sudden increase in venous pressure.

3. *Have there been previous episodes?*
Recurrence is common in all of the above conditions.

Eye examination

External

Ensure that there is no swelling of the lids or periorbital tissue (Plate 1), which may indicate orbital cellulitis (p. 150).

Visual acuity

Vision is unaffected in all of the above, although patients may complain of minimal reduction with severe conjunctivitis.

Conjunctiva

Look for a discharge indicating bacterial conjunctivitis.

A brick-red solid area of redness is typical of subconjunctival haemorrhage (Plate 3). Ask the patient to look down and identify the upper margin. Document this finding. If the upper margin is not visible, and trauma has occurred recently (usually head injury), the blood may have tracked forwards from an intracranial source, although this is extremely rare. The appearance may be alarming, with the conjunctiva prolapsing over the lower lid.

Sclera

A segmental area of inflammation over the white of the eye is indicative of episcleritis. This is an inflammation of the superficial layer of the sclera (episclera). There is no discharge, and the patient may complain of a slight irritation. Diffuse episcleritis may occur and may mimic conjunctivitis, but is not associated with a discharging or sticky eye and is frequently recurrent.

Cornea, pupil and fundus

The cornea, pupils and fundus are all normal.

Conjunctivitis

Features

The conjunctiva is usually diffusely red (Plate 2). Haemorrhages may be present. Conjunctivitis usually starts in one eye, prior to becoming bilateral. Discharge may be purulent in bacterial and watery in viral infection. Pain is unusual (p. 44), discomfort common.

Management

1. In severe cases take a bacterial swab, by asking the patient to look up, pulling down the lower lid, and sweeping the lower conjunctival fornix.
2. Stain the eye with dilute fluorescein and examine the cornea under a blue light to ensure that no corneal lesion is present, such as a dendritic ulcer (p. 27) or foreign body (p. 18), as these are not painful in all cases.
3. Discharge on chloramphenicol drops 0.5% 2-hourly for 2 days then q.d.s. for 8 days.
4. If treatment has already been started but has failed, take a swab and start on an alternative

antibiotic drop, such as gentamicin 0.3% (Genticin) 2-hourly, chloramphenicol 0.5% 2-hourly or fusidic acid ointment (Fucithalmic) 1% b.d. Ensure that the patient is in fact using the previous treatment and has done so for at least 3 days.

Referral

No referral is usually required. If treatment has failed after 10 days of adequate therapy, or pain or substantially reduced visual acuity are present, refer to the ophthalmologist within 24 hours.

Follow-up

Not required unless particularly severe, in which case review in 3 days. If worse, refer to the ophthalmologist within 24 hours rather than leaving for the above 10 days.

Subconjunctival haemorrhage

Features

Solid red discoloration (Plate 3), painless and frequently sharply demarcated. Usually idiopathic, but may follow a Valsalva manoeuvre.

Management

1. Identify the upper border of the haemorrhage and document this.
2. Check blood pressure (BP) and treat if required.
3. If there has been no history of ocular or head

trauma, reassure the patient that the haemorrhage will resolve spontaneously, but may take up to 6 weeks, and may initially worsen before improvement occurs.

4. No ocular treatment is necessary.

Referral

No referral is required for spontaneous subconjunctival haemorrhage provided there has been no related trauma (see Trauma, p. 116) and BP is normal.

Follow-up

No follow-up is required.

Pitfall

Identify and document that the upper border of the haemorrhage can be seen. Make the patient look down and lift the upper lid. If no border is visible following trauma, discuss with neurosurgeons – the blood may have tracked along the optic nerve from an intracranial source. The patient is likely to be unwell if this is the case.

Episcleritis

Features

Dilated vessels visible on the surface of the eye. There is not the solid red appearance typical of subconjunctival haemorrhage. Frequently medial or lateral aspect of eye affected.

Management

1. Stain the eye with fluorescein and examine for other lesions which cause a similar localized inflammation, such as marginal corneal ulcer (p. 27) or corneal foreign body (p. 18), as these may occasionally be painless.
2. If severely symptomatic, start on flurbiprofen (Froben) 100 mg b.d. p.o. for 2 weeks, provided there are no contraindications, such as peptic ulceration or concomitant anti-inflammatory treatment. The patient should be warned to stop treatment immediately and reattend should any gastric irritation occur.
3. Mild cases usually resolve spontaneously in 2–3 weeks and require no treatment.

Referral

Routine referral is not required. If the condition does not settle on the above treatment, refer to the ophthalmologist within 48 hours, as topical steroids may be required.

Follow-up

No follow-up is required.

Allergic reactions

See pp. 42, 57.

Red eye – acute, painless, bilateral

There are few causes of acute painless bilateral red eye.

Main causes

1. Conjunctivitis p. 50.
2. Blepharitis (inflammation of the lid margins with secondary ocular irritation) p. 56.
3. Allergic reactions p. 42.
4. Dysthyroid eye disease p. 47.

Relevant questions

1. *Is there a discharge?*
   Mucopurulent discharge is associated with bacterial conjunctivitis. Consider *Chlamydia* in the sexually active age group.
2. *Is the patient atopic?*
   These patients are prone to allergic reactions in response to numerous allergens, typically house dust or pollen.
3. *Is the patient on any treatment for thyroid disease, or are there symptoms or signs suggestive of hyperthyroidism?*
   Tremor, anxiety, temper, heat intolerance, palpitations, tachycardia or weight loss suggest thyroid overactivity. Although rare, bilateral red eyes may be the initial presentation of thyroid disease, and may be inappropriately treated as conjunctivitis.

Eye examination

External

Ensure that there is no swelling of the lids or

periorbital tissue (Plate 1) which would indicate orbital cellulitis (p. 150).

Visual acuity

Vision is usually unaffected in all of the above, although patients may complain of minimal reduction with severe conjunctivitis.

Conjunctiva

Look for a discharge indicating bacterial conjunctivitis. Pull down the lower lid and look at the lower conjunctiva in the gutter between the eye and the inner part of the lower lid (lower conjunctival fornix). Greyish translucent globules within the conjunctiva (best seen under a slitlamp) are associated with chlamydial infection, which should be suspected in the sexually active. Evert the upper lid (see Fig. 1.4, p. 7). A roughened injected undersurface occurs in allergic conjunctivitis.

Sclera

Injection over the medial and lateral aspect of the sclera may indicate thyroid eye disease, particularly if the eyes look prominent.

Cornea

Marginal corneal ulcers (p. 27) are associated with blepharitis (p. 56), and are not always painful. Stain the cornea with fluorescein and look for an ulcer. Diffuse staining may be related to exposure secondary to thyroid disease.

Pupils

An afferent pupillary defect (p. 3) may indicate optic nerve compression secondary to thyroid disease.

Fundus

Fundal appearances are usually normal.

Conjunctivitis

This is fully discussed on pp. 44, 50.

Blepharitis

Features

This is extremely common and is primarily an eyelid problem which leads to chronic bilateral ocular irritation (rather than pain) with acute exacerbations. The eyelashes may be matted, encrusted or have small flakes of adherent skin attached. The lid margin is frequently injected.

Management

1. Advise the patient that the condition is chronic and treatment is to relieve symptoms, but will not cure the underlying problem.
2. Stain the cornea with fluorescein to ensure that there is no associated corneal marginal ulcer (p. 27).
3. If the lids are very injected, start on chloramphenicol ointment 1% t.d.s. The patient should firmly

rub this into the eyelid margins, at the base of the eyelashes for 3 weeks. There is no need to instil this into the eye.

4. Lid hygiene. Advise the patient to clean the lid margins thoroughly morning and night by pulling the skin of the outer lid margins laterally to put the lids under tension. With a clean lint cloth or flannel dampened with a mild solution of saline (one teaspoon of salt in a tumbler of cooled boiled water) or baby shampoo, firmly rub the margins to remove grease and debris associated with the condition. This treatment should be continued indefinitely.

Referral

Not required in the absence of corneal pathology. If corneal staining is present, refer to the ophthalmologist within 24 hours.

Follow-up

Not required other than by the ophthalmologist if the patient is referred as above.

Allergic reactions

Features

Not uncommon in children who may rub an allergen into their eyes. Frequently occurs as a result of exposure to dust, fur or pollen in atopic individuals, antibiotic eye drops, make-up or contact lens solution. Presentation varies from virtually no injection at all, to erythematous, oedematous sticky red eyes and surrounding skin.

Management

1. If erythema or inflammation of the lids or periorbital tissues is present, treat as periorbital or orbital cellulitis (p. 151).
2. If the lids or periorbital tissues are simply swollen but not injected, this is typical of an acute allergic response, particularly if the conjunctiva is similarly swollen (it may appear as a pale yellow coloured bag of fluid surrounding the cornea). Antihistamines may be given orally. However, the condition usually resolves rapidly without these.
3. Identify any possible allergen from the history.
4. Stop any antibiotic eye drops, and do not substitute another.
5. If the patient is a contact lens wearer, these should be removed, and left out until reviewed as below.
6. Advise the patient to stop using make-up, or change to a hypoallergenic variety.
7. Cold compresses are useful. Advise the patient to soak a clean flannel in cold water and place over the closed eyes.
8. Do not treat with eye drops or ointment, as these may exacerbate the problem.

Referral

Orbital or periorbital cellulitis – ophthalmology opinion immediately.
Children with swollen (but not injected) lids – discuss with ophthalmologist. Settles within 24 hours.

Contact lens wear or antibiotic drops – ophthalmology opinion within 24 hours.
All other cases – discharge.

Follow-up

This is required only in cases that have not settled within 24 hours, and these should be referred to the ophthalmologist within 24 hours of their return to the surgery or casualty.

Dysthyroid eye disease

This is fully discussed on p. 47.

Red eye – chronic, unilateral or bilateral

Main causes

1. Blepharitis
2. Chronic conjunctivitis
3. Contact lens wear
4. Dry eye
5. Dysthyroid eye disease

Relevant questions

1. *Does the patient get crusting of the eyelids, or stuck-down lids in the morning?*
   This is typical of blepharitis (p. 56).
2. *Does the patient have arthritis?*
   Dry eye is common in the elderly and those with rheumatoid arthritis (p. 61).

3. *Does he or she wear contact lenses?*
   Lens intolerance and poor lens hygeine should be considered (p. 135).
4. *Is there a discharge?*
   Chronic conjunctivitis is a less common cause of chronic red eye (pp. 44, 50).
5. *Is the problem work-related?*
   Does the patient work in a dry dusty atmosphere?
6. *Is there a history of thyroid disease?*
   This is commonly treated as chronic conjunctivitis until properly diagnosed (p. 47).

Eye examination

External

Look for the staring appearance associated with thyroid eye disease, particularly if the eyes look prominent.

Lids

Bilateral red lid margins, and lashes that are matted together or scattered with dry skin debris is typical of blepharitis. Chronic unilateral blepharitis in an elderly patient may represent a rare form of lid tumour (sebaceous gland carcinoma). A small elevated lesion on the lid margin, similar to a viral wart, may cause a unilateral chronic irritable eye, usually in children (molluscum contagiosum).

Conjunctiva

A suffused-looking conjunctiva is common in chronic alcohol abuse. Consider chronic conjunctivitis if a discharge is present, and *Chlamydia* in the sexually active. Dry eyes lead to debris in the tear film and loss of tear meniscus between lower lid and globe (best seen on a slitlamp). Fluorescein highlights these features.

Cornea

Dry eyes may lead to corneal exposure, which stains diffusely with fluorescein. Patients typically describe a gritty sensation.

If vision is reduced, check the fundus for any gross abnormalities. Reduced vision is discussed on p. 63.

Features, management and follow-up

Blepharitis is dealt with on p. 56.
Conjunctivitis is dealt with on pp. 44, 50.
Thyroid eye disease is dealt with on p. 47.
Contact lens problems are dealt with on p. 135.

Dry eye

Features

Gritty eyes which may be diffusely red. Common in the elderly and those with rheumatoid arthritis.

Management

1. Stain the cornea with fluorescein, and observe under a blue light. Diffuse areas of fine punctate staining indicates dry eyes.

2. Start on hypromellose 0.3% drops every 2 hours and Lacri-Lube ointment at night.

Referral

All patients demonstrating corneal staining with fluorescein should be reviewed at an early ophthalmology outpatient clinic once treatment has been initiated as above. If the cornea is clear, no referral is required.

Follow-up

Not required other than by the ophthalmologist if the patient is referred as above.

3 Visual symptoms

The most common visual complaints are:
1. Loss of vision below
2. Floaters, flashes and 'cobwebs' p. 95
3. Double vision p. 96.

Loss of vision

Reduced visual acuity or loss of visual field

Which category applies?
Acute unilateral visual loss p. 66
Acute bilateral visual loss p. 84
Chronic unilateral or bilateral visual loss p. 88
Transient loss of vision p. 92.

Relevant questions

1. *Is visual loss acute or chronic, unilateral or bilateral?*
Acute conditions tend to be unilateral, chronic ones bilateral

Acute loss occurs in retinal artery (Plate 13) or vein occlusion (Plate 7), haemorrhage at the macula (usually a spontaneous event in the elderly), ischaemia of the optic nerve, retinal detachment and vitreous haemorrhage.

Chronic visual loss is usually secondary to cataract, age-related degeneration of the retina in the elderly, chronic glaucoma, or the patient may simply be wearing old glasses. It is rarely due to retinal detachment or intraocular tumour.

2. *Is loss of visual acuity total or just blurred?* *Sudden total loss* (vision of hand movements, perception of light or less) without pain indicates retinal arterial occlusion (usually 65+ years) or optic nerve ischaemia (45+ years; see Fig. 1.5a, p. 8) Less profound, sudden painless visual loss occurs in retinal vein occlusion (40+ age group) and vitreous haemorrhage (any age).
3. *Is field loss central, peripheral or altitudinal (upper or lower half)?*
   Field loss can occur in the presence of normal visual acuity.
4. *Central visual field loss* (see Fig. 1.5b, p. 8) occurs in optic neuritis (20–40-year age group), age-related retinal degeneration and macular haemorrhage (60+ age group).
5. *Peripheral field loss* may occur in glaucoma, retinal detachment or following a stroke which affects the visual pathway. The latter leads to field loss which will vary according to the site affected, but is usually behind the optic chiasm and therefore affects either the left or right hemifield of vision (i.e. both left-hand sides of vision of each eye or right-hand sides – homonymous hemianopia, see Fig. 1.5c, p.8).

   Remember that bilateral temporal field loss (see Fig. 1.5d, p. 8) indicates a tumour in the region of the optic chiasm until otherwise proven, particularly in the presence of optic disc pallor. The patient may complain of 'bumping into things' to the side.
6. *Altitudinal field loss* (see Fig. 1.5e, p. 8) is typical of optic nerve ischaemia, particularly in hypertensives (45+ years).

7. *Floaters or flashing lights prior to field loss* (p. 95)? Look for evidence of retinal detachment (p. 79).
8. *Is it painful?* Trauma, endophthalmitis (infection within the eye) and acute glaucoma are painful, whereas most other causes of visual loss are painless. Haloes may be seen around lights in glaucoma.
9. *Has there been any trauma?*
   (a) *Acute trauma* – go to p. 116.
   (b) *Old trauma* – retinal detachment may follow old trauma and is often associated with floaters and flashes (p. 95).
10. *Is the patient hypertensive?* This is the most common underlying cause of retinal vein occlusion and ischaemic damage to the optic nerve. Arteriosclerosis predisposes to retinal artery occlusion by direct occlusion or via emboli thrown off from the carotids.
11. *Is there any evidence of temporal arteritis?* Malaise, shoulder girdle pain, scalp tenderness, weight loss, jaw claudication with eating and headaches all point to this diagnosis in the over-55s. Optic nerve ischaemia or retinal artery occlusion may rapidly involve both eyes if untreated.
12. *Is the patient diabetic?* Vitreous haemorrhage may occur in diabetics with proliferative retinopathy. This may rarely be the presenting feature of diabetes.
13. *Has the patient had any previous eye surgery?* Recent surgery (2–14 days) combined with a painful eye and visual loss indicates endophthalmitis (infection of the interior of the eye) until otherwise proven. Retinal detachment may recur following previous detachment surgery for this condition, or following cataract extraction.

Acute unilateral visual loss

See 'Relevant questions' on p. 63.

Main causes

1. Central retinal artery occlusion (CRAO, Plate 13)	painless p. 69
2. Anterior ischaemic optic neuropathy (AION, Plate 6) secondary to:	
(a) *Temporal arteritis*	headaches p. 72
(b) *Arteriosclerosis*	painless p. 73
3. Central retinal vein occlusion (Plate 7)	painless p. 74
4. Macular haemorrhage (disciform)	painless p. 75
5. Trauma	± pain p. 116

Less common causes

1. Endophthalmitis	painful pp. 167–171
2. Acute glaucoma	painful p. 30
3. Optic neuritis	± pain p. 76
4. Vitreous haemorrhage	painless p. 78
5. Retinal detachment	painless p. 79
6. Functional	painless p. 82

Eye examination

External

Externally the eye is usually normal.

Trauma should be apparent from the history.

Red eye – consider acute glaucoma in the elderly or endophthalmitis if previous eye surgery has been undertaken. Iritis may lead to a moderate reduction in vision rather than severe loss, and is associated with photophobia (pain looking at light).

Pupils

Afferent pupil defect (poor response to direct light, but brisk when a light is shone in the normal eye (p. 3) is present in CRAO, optic neuritis and in some cases of CRVO and retinal detachment. In acute glaucoma it may be semidilated and sluggish.

Eye movements

If painful, consider optic neuritis.

Fields

If there is any remaining vision at all, cover the good eye and make the patient look at one of your eyes. Move a finger in from the side from all four quadrants approximately 30 cm in front of the patient's eye and observe any missing field. There may only be loss of central field (optic neuritis, age-related retinal degeneration). This field test is crude, but all that is required in a casualty setting. Compare perception of a bright red object between the two eyes, as colour desaturation indicates optic nerve disease (optic neuritis).

Conjunctiva

This may be markedly swollen in trauma and endophthalmitis, but is normal in most other cases of acute visual loss.

Cornea

The cornea is usually normal; however, a hazy cornea in association with a painful red eye and reduced vision is characteristic of acute glaucoma in the elderly.

Anterior chamber

Naked-eye examination may reveal a hypopyon (pus in the anterior chamber which settles as a whitish level at the base of the cornea, Plate 9). This is in keeping with endophthalmitis or severe uveitis and is best seen with a slitlamp. A hazy view of the iris may be secondary to corneal oedema as a result of acute glaucoma (p. 30).

Lens

Cataract may present as an acute problem. Ask if the patient only noticed the problem when he or she covered the good eye.

Fundus

Examination often reveals the diagnosis.
Pale fundus – often with a reddish spot at the macula – indicates a CRAO (Plate 13). Look at the arteries and veins carefully – you may see red blood cells sluggishly flowing through them. Look for emboli blocking the arteries. These appear as white flecks in the vessel lumen and indicate carotid disease (listen to the carotids for bruits).
Swollen optic disc (Plate 6) – consider AION – compare this with the other disc. If both are swollen, this is papilloedema until proven otherwise.

Retrobulbar neuritis does not usually cause disc swelling, as the affected part of the optic nerve is posterior to the optic disc.
Retinal haemorrhages – in a sector of retina (Plate 7) or widely distributed, indicate retinal vein occlusion. Disc swelling may be present. Ensure this is not diabetic retinopathy – look for similar changes in the other eye and check the urine.
Macular haemorrhage – commonly associated with preceding age-related maculopathy (ARM). Look in the unaffected eye – macular degeneration (mottled pigmented appearance) is often present.
Difficult or hazy view – may be due to a small pupil or cataract. Consider vitreous haemorrhage, particularly if dark strands can be seen behind the lens and the patient is diabetic. Look at the red reflex; this is the reflection through the pupil when observed through an ophthalmoscope 30 cm or so from the patient. Loss of this reflex indicates vitreous opacity (blood) but can occur in dense cataract or corneal opacity.

Central retinal artery occlusion (CRAO)

Features

Painless, profound sudden visual loss, afferent pupil defect, pale fundus with a red spot at the central macula (cherry-red spot, Plate 13). Recovery is unlikely, particularly if over 6 hours from onset.

Associations

Arteriosclerosis, temporal arteritis, carotid disease, atrial fibrillation, migraine (very rare).

Management

1. Consider temporal arteritis (p. 72). Take blood for erythrocyte sedimentation rate (ESR).
   A normal ESR does not exclude temporal arteritis.
2. Try to re-establish arterial flow by lowering intraocular pressure (IOP) and dilating retinal arterioles as follows:
   (a) Give i.v. Diamox (acetazolamide) 500 mg stat (lowers IOP).
   (b) Give sublingual GTN 300 μg (dilates arteries).
   (c) Massage the eye. Lie the patient down, and tell him or her to look towards their feet. Stand behind the patient, and with both of your index fingers, ballot the globe firmly through the patient's eyelids. Do this firmly – if it is not uncomfortable for the patient, you are not massaging effectively. Continue for 5–10 minutes, releasing intermittently.
   (d) Get the patient to breathe in and out from a medium-sized paper bag. This raises $P\text{co}_2$ and dilates the arteries.
3. Give hydrocortisone 200 mg i.v. stat only if the history and examination suggest temporal arteritis (60+ years old, temporal or occipital headache, malaise, weight loss, scalp tenderness, jaw pain with eating or tender, nodular, poorly pulsatile temporal arteries, raised ESR) and admit under the ophthalmologists or physicians for oral steroids 80–120 mg p.o. enteric coated initially for 3 days and reduced slowly thereafter or pulsed i.v. methyl prednisolone. Take the usual precautions before starting high-dose steroids in hypertensives and those with a history of peptic ulceration. Cover this latter group with ranitidine (Zantac) 150 mg b.d. p.o.

4. Start aspirin 75 mg p.o. o.d. if arteriosclerotic with no evidence of temporal arteritis, and no contra-indications to aspirin.

Referral

- If under 12 hours from onset, treat as above and refer to the ophthalmologists immediately.
- If over 12 hours from onset but temporal arteritis suspected, treat as above and refer immediately to ophthalmologist. There is a high risk of the other eye becoming involved.
- If over 12 hours old, ESR and BP normal and no evidence of temporal arteritis, discuss with ophthalmologist prior to review within 12–24 hours.
- If BP raised, or carotid bruits/heart murmurs present, but no evidence of temporal arteritis – refer to physicians or vascular surgeons as appropriate (for carotid Doppler scan) in addition to ophthalmology review within 24 hours. The ophthalmologist may arrange vascular specialist referral.

Follow-up

Ophthalmologist will arrange this.

Pitfall

Always consider temporal arteritis, even if the ESR is normal, as failure to adequately treat this condition may lead to loss of vision in the other eye within hours or days.

Anterior ischaemic optic neuropathy (AION)

There are two main categories of AION:

1. *Temporal arteritis (arteritic)* – blockage of the arteries supplying the optic nerve secondary to arterial inflammation.
2. *Arteriosclerotic (non-arteritic)* – blockage due to atherosclerotic arteriolar narrowing.

• Temporal arteritis

Features

Age group 60+, headache, malaise, scalp tenderness, jaw claudication, shoulder girdle myalgia, weight loss, transient diplopia, palpable nodular tender temporal arteries. These signs and symptoms frequently precede profound visual loss with an afferent pupil defect (p. 3) and a swollen pale optic disc.

Associations

Polymyalgia rheumatica, idiopathic.

Management

1. Take an ESR.
2. Give hydrocortisone 200 mg i.v. stat.
3. Admit under the ophthalmologists or physicians for oral steroids, 80–120 mg p.o. enteric coated initially for 3 days and reduced slowly thereafter, or pulsed i.v. methyl prednisolone. Take the usual precautions before starting high-dose steroids in hypertensives and those with a history of peptic

Plate 1

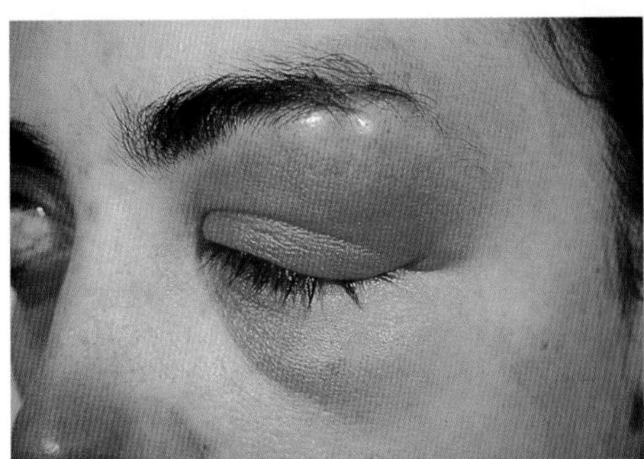

Orbital cellulitis. Traumatic periorbital swelling and erythema may appear similar.

Plate 2

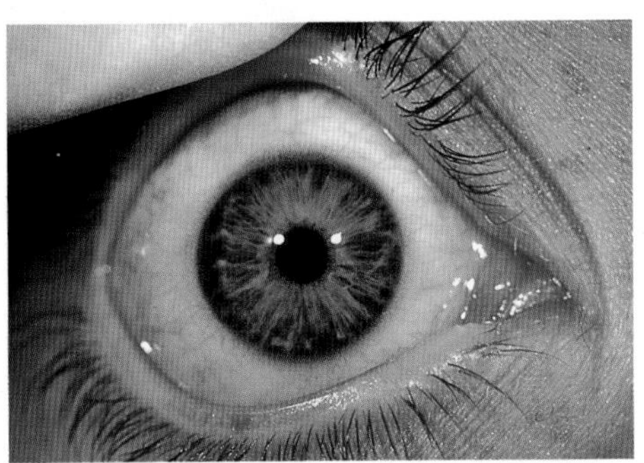

Mild bacterial conjunctivitis. If painful, consider iritis.

Plate 3

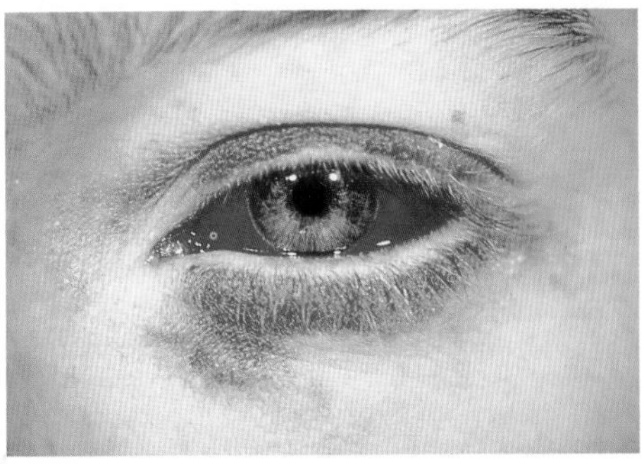

Posttraumatic periorbital bruising and subconjunctival haemorrhage.

Plate 4

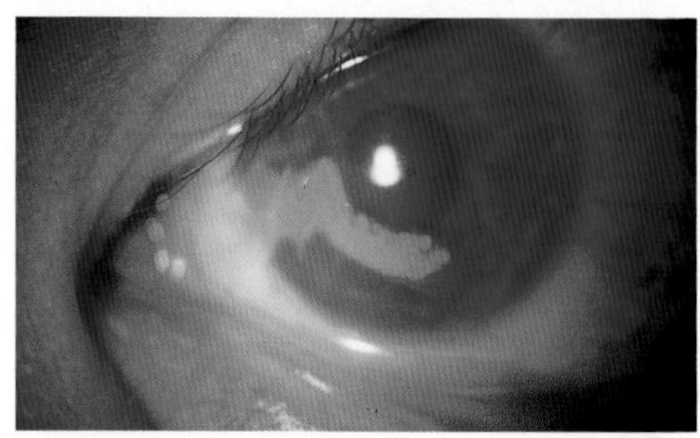

Corneal abrasion highlighted by staining with fluorescein and observed under a blue light.

Plate 5

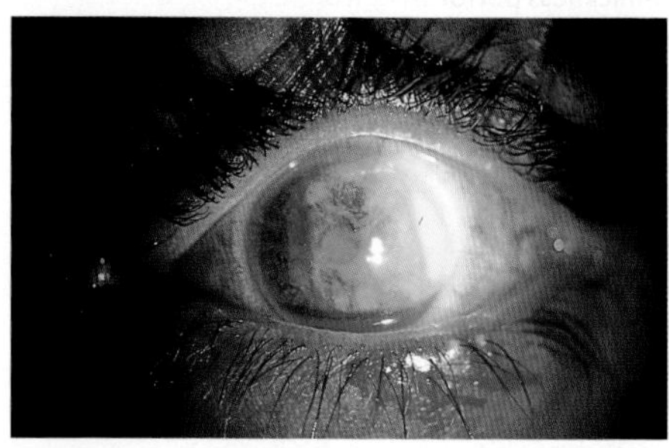

Upper corneal scratches associated with subtarsal foreign body.

Plate 6
Plate 7

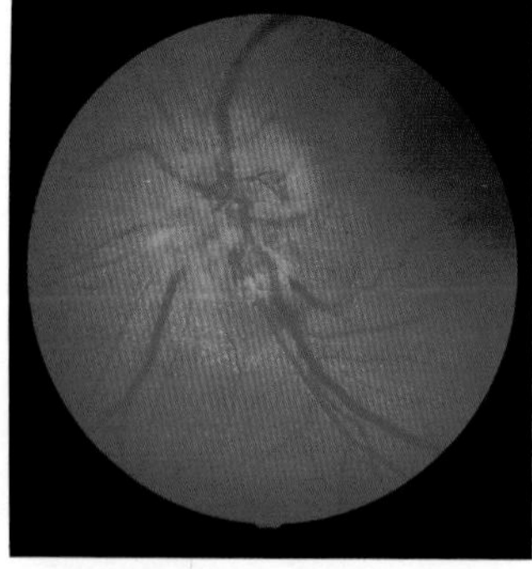

Swollen optic disc with haemorrhages. Consider anterior ischaemic optic neuropathy (see under temporal arteritis), central retinal vein occlusion and papilloedema (usually bilateral).

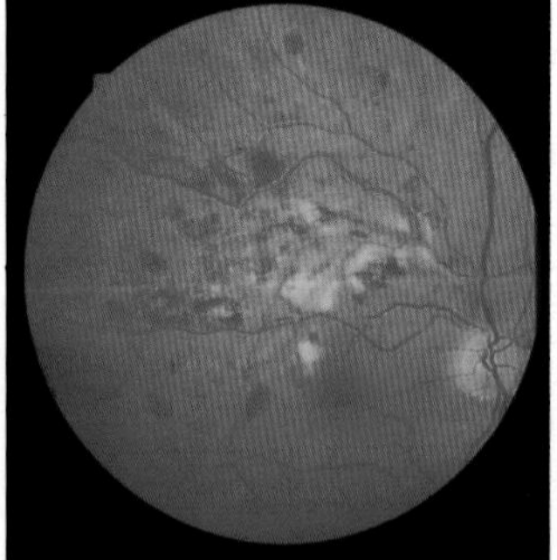

Branch retinal vein occlusion with multiple haemorrhages and cotton-wool spots. Note that only one quadrant is affected. If the appearance is more widespread and bilateral, consider diabetic retinopathy.

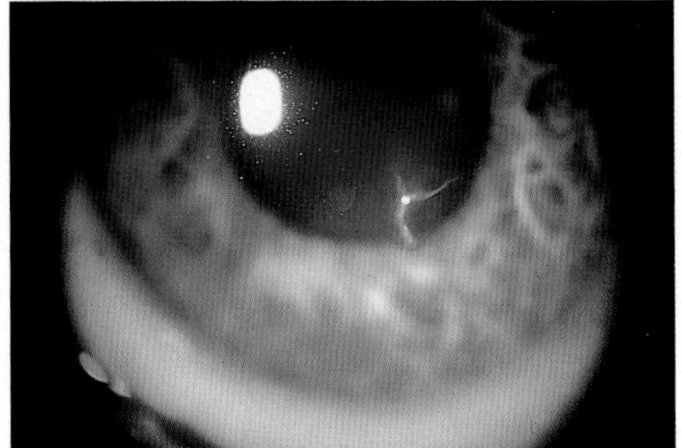

Plate 8

Full-thickness perforating wound of the cornea.

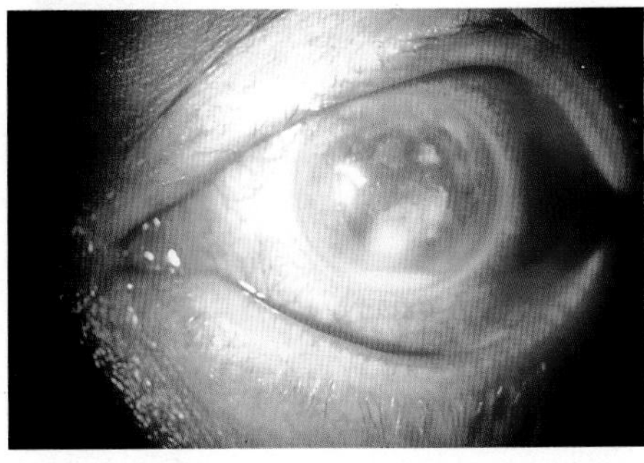

Plate 9

Bacterial keratitis. Corneal ulcer with corneal abscess and hypopyon. Consider endophthalmitis if after trauma or surgery.

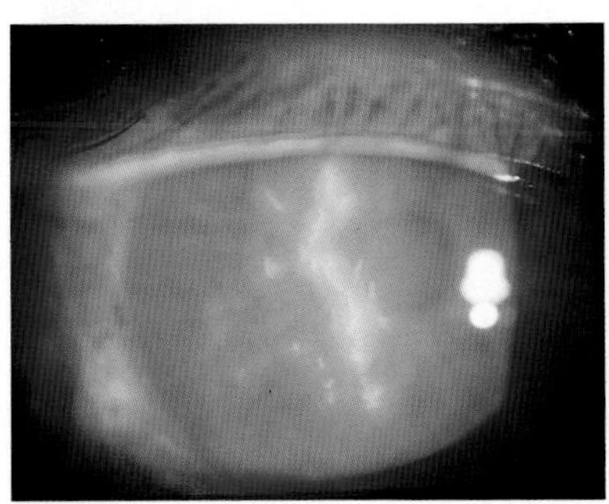

Plate 10

Dendritic (branching) herpes simplex corneal ulcer.

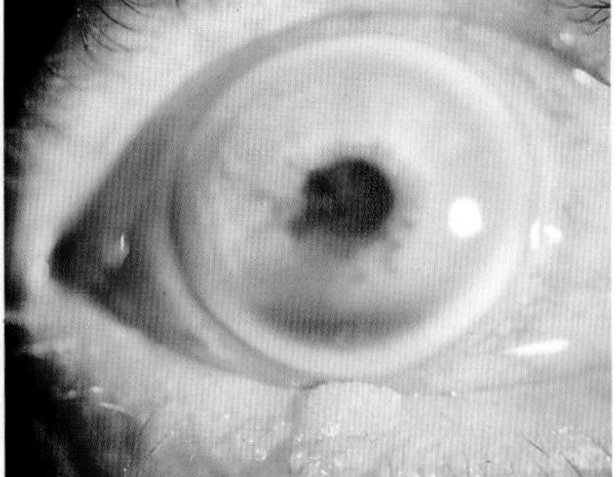

Plate 11

Hyphaema.

Plate 12

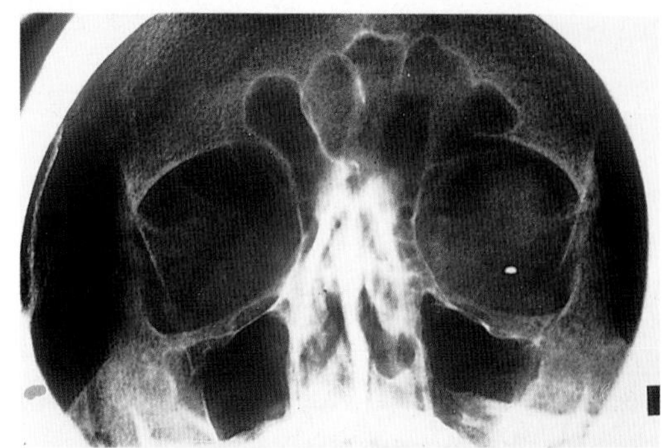

Radiopaque intraocular foreign body. Lateral view should also be obtained.

Plate 13

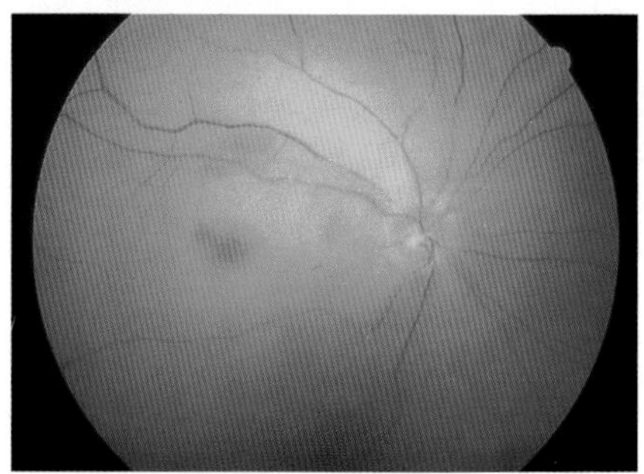

Central retinal artery occlusion. The infarcted retina is pale and oedematous. There is a classical cherry-red spot at the macula.

Plate 14

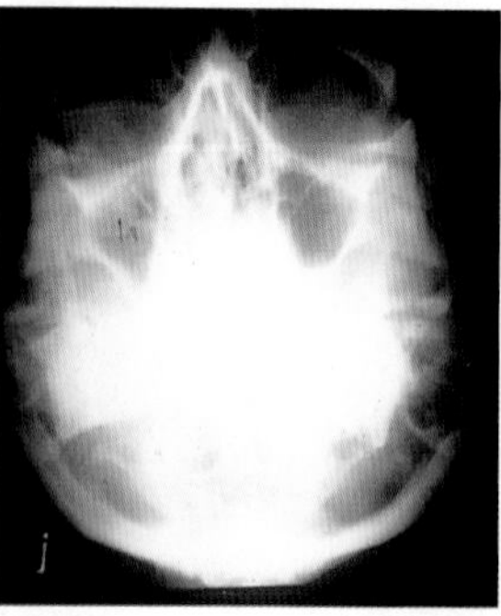

Blow-out fracture. Note maxillary sinus opacification due to prolapsed orbital tissue. Sinusitis may appear similar.

ulceration. Cover this latter group with ranitidine (Zantac) 150 mg b.d. p.o.

4. Measure BP and treat as required.

Referral

Immediately to the ophthalmologist. Admit as above for high-dose steroids, either under the ophthalmologists or physicians. There is a high risk of permanent blindness in the unaffected eye without prompt adequate treatment.

Follow-up

Ophthalmologist only.

• Arteriosclerotic (non-arteritic)

Features

Age group 45+. Visual loss is frequently less profound compared with temporal arteritis. Altitudinal field loss is common, that is, loss of upper or lower half of field (see Fig. 1.5, p. 8). Pale swollen optic disc, afferent pupil defect.

Management

1. Suspect temporal arteritis. Take an ESR. If raised (usually over 60 s) treat as temporal arteritis, even in the absence of other symptoms. A normal ESR does not rule out temporal arteritis.

2. Check BP. Hypertension is the most common underlying cause of non-arteritic AION.
3. Check urine and random blood for diabetes.
4. Listen to carotids for bruits and heart sounds for murmurs.
5. Start on aspirin 75 mg p.o. o.d if there are no contraindications to this, and there is no evidence of temporal arteritis.
6. Strongly advise the patient to stop smoking.

Referral

Discuss immediately with the ophthalmologist. Uncontrolled hypertension should be discussed with the physicians.

Follow-up

Ophthalmologist only.

Central retinal vein occlusion or branch vein occlusion

If only part of the retinal venous system is occluded, the condition is called a branch retinal vein occlusion, and fundal signs occur only in that sector (Plate 7).

Features

Moderate to marked sudden painless visual loss, afferent pupil defect in severe cases only, retinal haemorrhages, which may be few in number or widespread, occasionally cotton-wool spots (patchy white retinal lesions related to ischaemia) and disc swelling (Plate 6).

Associations

Hypertension is by far the most common association. Smoking, glaucoma (raised eye pressure), diabetes, raised blood viscosity (multiple myeloma, polycythaemia).

Management

1. Measure BP and treat as required.
2. Check urine and random blood for diabetes.
3. Send blood for full blood count, plasma electrophoresis, blood sugar and cholesterol.
4. Strongly advise the patient to stop smoking.

Referral

All cases should be referred to the ophthalmologist within 48 hours for measurement of intra-ocular pressure (IOP).

Follow-up

Ophthalmologist will arrange this.

Macular haemorrhage

Features

Usual age group 65+. Central visual loss (see Fig. 1.5b, p. 8) with normal peripheral vision. Patient describes difficulty in reading and recognizing people. Painless. Frequently preceded by distortion – typically straight lines appear wavy or have bits missing.

Management

There is no immediate management appropriate to casualty or general practice.

Referral

Profound loss

Refer to the ophthalmology outpatient department routinely. There is no useful treatment at this stage. Ask about visual distortion in the other eye – see below.

Visual distortion or blurring

Discuss immediately with the ophthalmologist. On rare occasions, laser treatment can arrest progression to profound loss.

Follow-up

Ophthalmology outpatient department only.

Optic neuritis (ON)

Features

Age group 20–40 years, central visual loss (although vision may be normal), reduction in colour perception (particularly red), reduction in light brightness perception (light is brighter in normal eye), afferent pupil defect (p. 3), discomfort with eye movements, discomfort if globe is gently pressed over closed eyelid, normal disc and retina.

Associations

Idiopathic is by far the most common. Postviral (usually upper respiratory tract infection) in children. Although multiple sclerosis is associated with ON, a single episode is not sufficient for this diagnosis to be made and should not be given to the patient unless you are questioned on this topic. To do so causes unjustified concern to the patient. If there is a previous history of neurological dysfunction – characteristically limb paraesthesia and weakness, or previous optic neuritis – then demyelinating disease should be suspected.

Management

1. There is no acute management appropriate in a GP or emergency room setting. Do not give steroids unless advised to do so.
2. Document the visual acuity in each eye with glasses, if worn.
3. Look for an afferent pupil defect (p. 3), which is usually present.
4. Enquire about previous neurological events.

Referral

Discuss all cases with the ophthalmologist within 24 hours. He or she will arrange neurology referral if required.

Follow-up

Ophthalmology or neurology outpatient department only.

Vitreous haemorrhage

Features

Moderate to profound visual loss which is painless and usually preceded by floaters, 'cobwebs' or flashes in vision (p. 95) with no afferent pupil defect. There is usually poor or absent visibility of the retina, with loss of the red reflex.

Associations

Diabetes, old retinal vein occlusion, torn retinal blood vessel secondary to posterior vitreous detachment (detachment of the vitreous jelly from its normal retinal attachments, Fig. 3.1, p. 81) and trauma.

Management

1. If related to trauma, check for other non-ocular trauma and fully examine the eye and orbit as described on p. 118.
2. Check urine and send off a random blood sugar if the patient is not a known diabetic.
3. Look at the fundus of the other eye for retinal haemorrhages which may indicate diabetic retinopathy.

Referral

All traumatic cases should be discussed with the ophthalmologist immediately. All other cases should be referred within 24 hours, with the exception of known diabetics with recurrent vitreous haemorrhages who only require to be referred to an early (few days) ophthalmology clinic and advised not to undertake any strenuous activity. New diabetics should be discussed with the physicians and seen within 24 hours by the ophthalmologist.

Follow-up

Ophthalmologist – who will arrange for further referral to the physicians in the case of new diabetics.

Pitfalls

Failure to examine opposite eye for retinal pathology. Proliferative retinopathy which requires urgent treatment may be present.

Retinal detachment

Features

Often preceded by 'flashes', 'cobwebs' or a shower of floaters in visual field (p. 95). Loss of part or all of the visual field which is painless and may progress over several days. Often described as a shutter or curtain coming down over the eye. Visual distortion rather than visual loss may occur. An afferent pupil defect

(p. 3) may be present in a large detachment. Fundal examination may reveal greyish-coloured mobile retina, sometimes with a rippled surface; however in long-standing cases the retina may be almost translucent and difficult to visualize.

Associations

Myopia (short-sightedness – look through the patient's glasses – a myopic correction makes objects look smaller), torn retina secondary to posterior vitreous detachment (detachment of the vitreous jelly from its normal retinal attachments, Fig. 3.1), trauma, which need not be recent and is often blunt in nature, previous eye surgery for detached retina or cataract, idiopathic.

Management

1. Document visual acuity.
2. If there is a history of recent trauma, examine for other ocular (p. 116) and non-ocular injuries.
3. On fundoscopy, attempt to see if the macula (the part of the retina just temporal to the optic disc) is still attached. If the visual acuity is 6/12 or better, it most probably is attached.

Referral

Discuss all cases with the ophthalmologist immediately. Fresh detachments should be admitted under the ophthalmologists, particularly if the visual acuity is still good. Old detachments (over 1 week),

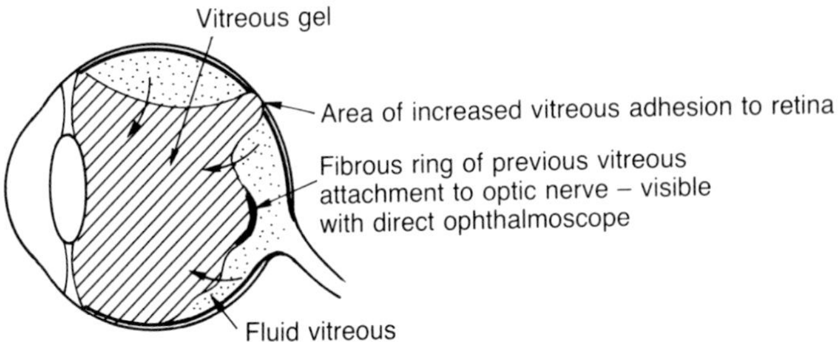

(a) Vitreous gel peels away from its retinal attachments

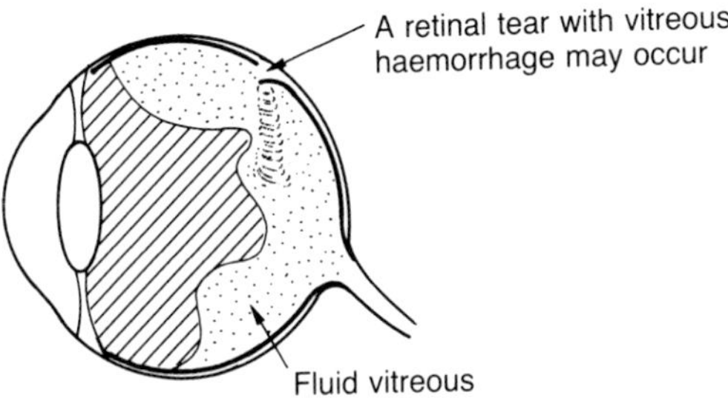

(b) Vitreous gel fully detaches

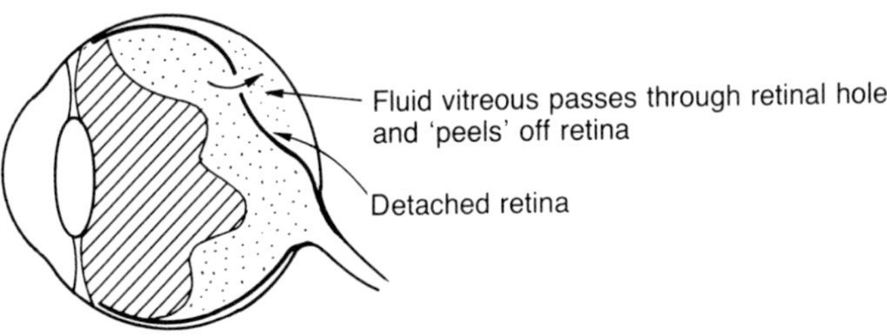

(c) Retinal detachment

Fig. 3.1. (a) Posterior vitreous detachment; (b) retinal tear and (c) retinal detachment.

particularly those with poor visual acuity, should be assessed within 24–48 hours by the ophthalmologist.

Follow-up

Ophthalmologist only.

Pitfall

Failure to refer if there is a suspicion of retinal detachment may result in a simple detachment becoming complicated with a worse prognosis.

Functional loss

This relates to patients complaining of visual loss for which no cause can be found.

Features

Symptoms and signs which do not fit. The patient is often quite unconcerned. Bizarre field defects. 'Blind' patients may still navigate around the examining room with little difficulty, or wince at a bright light.

Associations

Attention-seeking, hysteria, malingering, psychiatric disturbance. Malingering is frequently associated with compensation claims. Hysterical loss is common in adolescent girls and children with home or schooling problems.

Management

1. Document visual acuity in each eye individually, with glasses if these are worn.
2. Document pupil reactions (normal in functional loss) and visual fields (pp. 7–9).
3. Shine a *bright* light into each eye and observe whether the patient blinks in the 'blind' eye.
4. Document fundal findings. Pay particular attention to the optic disc, which should be pink and healthy, and the macula (the retina temporal to the disc) which should have a flat appearance, with a small light reflex over its central part.
5. Functional loss is less likely in the elderly – consider an occipital infarct which has destroyed the visual cortex, particularly if there is a history of cardiovascular disease. Pupils will be normal in an occipital infarct.

Referral

All cases should be discussed with the ophthalmologist immediately. Functional loss is a diagnosis of exclusion, and requires detailed tests to confirm. On occasions, true pathology may appear to be functional.

Follow-up

Ophthalmologist only, who will refer further if required.

Acute bilateral visual loss

Acute bilateral visual loss is rarely attributable to ocular disease, but usually occurs as a result of vascular disease affecting the visual pathways.

Main cause

Arteriosclerosis resulting in:

1. Vertebral artery insufficiency
2. Occipital ischaemia or stroke
3. Optic nerve ischaemia (AION) – consider temporal arteritis

Less common causes

1. Functional or hysterical – often in children or compensation-related cases
2. Proliferative diabetic retinopathy
3. Blood dyscrasias leading to bilateral central retinal vein occlusion (CRVO)
4. Malignant hypertension
5. Migraine (see p. 110)

Relevant questions

1. *How long has visual loss been present for?*
   If visual loss was transient (see p. 92), consider vascular insufficiency, temporal arteritis, papilloedema or embolic disease secondary to arteriosclerosis.

2. *Is there a history of cardiovascular disease or diabetes?*
   Ask about angina, previous heart attack, hypertension, strokes or diabetes.
3. *Is there associated pain?*
   A frontal headache may be associated with migraine, temporal arteritis or an occipital infarct. If associated with scalp tenderness, jaw claudication, myalgia and malaise, temporal arteritis is likely (p. 72). A sharp occipital headache with visual loss in a conscious patient may represent a small subarachnoid bleed. A larger bleed is unlikely to present as an ophthalmological problem initially.
4. *Does the patient smoke or drink heavily?*
   Subacute bilateral profound visual loss can occur in this group, particularly if associated with a poor diet (tobacco/alcohol and nutritional amblyopias).
5. *Has there been a history of head injury in recent weeks?*
   A subdural haemorrhage may compress the occipital cortex.

Eye examination

External

Usually normal.

Visual acuity

Variable. Profound loss occurs in AION. In CRVO loss may be moderate or profound. Central acuity may be preserved in an occipital infarct and is usually normal in all but the late stages of papilloedema.

Fields

Bilateral symmetrical (congruous) peripheral and central field loss is typical of an occipital infarct. Total or altitudinal field loss (superior or inferior half of field; see Fig. 1.5e, p. 8) occurs in AION. Bizarre or inconsistant field loss is associated with functional loss.

Pupils

Sluggish light reaction in each pupil if bilateral AION (but response to accommodation is normal). Pupil responses are normal in occipital infarct and functional loss. Use a bright light source and observe if the patient blinks. This will occur in functional blindness if the patient is not prepared for this test.

Fundi

Disc swelling, haemorrhages and cotton-wool spots (Plate 6) are associated with CRVO, AION and papilloedema. If occipital pain is present, suspect a small subarachnoid haemorrhage.

Normal disc appearance is consistant with occipital infarct and functional loss. An embolus (white plaque seen in the vessel lumen) may be present at the disc, and if this has led to an arterial occlusion, the retina supplied by this vessel will appear pale. A cherry-red spot may be seen at the macula in the acute stage (Plate 13). Bilateral simultaneous loss due to emboli is extremely rare.

Retinal haemorrhages and cotton-wool spots occur in diabetes and CRVO. Bilateral CRVO is rare. It is associated with hypertension, raised IOP and blood dyscrasias such as polycythaemia and multiple myeloma.

General examination

Check BP, urinalysis, carotids for bruits and heart sounds for murmurs.

Observe how patients navigate around the room – are they as blind as they claim? Ask them to write their names on a piece of paper – truly blind people will have no problem with this.

Management

All cases should be discussed immediately with the ophthalmologist.

1. Always consider temporal arteritis (p. 72), particularly in AION or CRAO.
2. Check BP, full blood count, plasma proteins and cholesterol, if retinal vein occlusion is suspected (Plate 7). An ophthalmology opinion within 24 hours is required. Treat BP if elevated and consult with physicians if necessary.
3. Acute papilloedema is usually associated with normal visual acuity, in comparison to profound loss with AION. It requires urgent neurosurgical referral, as does suspected subarachnoid haemorrhage.
4. Suspected occipital infarct may require confirmation with computed tomography scan after discussing with the neurologists.
5. Suspected functional loss should be initially discussed with the ophthalmologist, followed within 24 hours by an ophthalmological assessment. Patients may be very convincing.
6. Aspirin 75 mg p.o. o.d. if a carotid bruit or heart

murmur is present and there are no contraindications to aspirin.
7. Advise the patient to stop drinking alcohol and smoking.

Referral

Discuss all cases with the ophthalmologist immediately.
Carotid bruits – discuss with vascular surgeons, who will advise on Doppler scan assessment of carotids.
Heart murmurs and uncontrolled hypertension – physicians.

Follow-up

Ophthalmologist/referred specialist only.

Chronic unilateral and bilateral visual loss

Main causes

1. ARM (age related maculopathy). This is an age-related degeneration of the central retina.
2. Cataract.
3. Incorrect or old glasses.

Most patients with cataract and age-related macular degeneration are aged 70 or more.

Less common causes

1. Glaucoma, hypertension and diabetes.
2. Space-occupying lesion.
3. Heavy consumption of alcohol and cigarettes.
4. Keratoconus.

Pain is not usually a feature of chronic bilateral visual loss.

Relevant questions

1. *For how long has deterioration been occurring?* Cataract and ARM can occur over months or years.
2. *How old are their present glasses?* They may require new glasses if these are over 2 years old.
3. *Is it just reading that the patient finds difficult?* This may be onset of presbyopia (difficulty with reading) if the patient is aged 40–50.
4. *Does the patient suffer from glaucoma, diabetes or hypertension?* Glaucoma may slowly destroy the optic nerve. Diabetes and hypertension may lead to retinal oedema with loss of vision.
5. *Does the patient drink or smoke heavily?* Nutritional and toxic amblyopia can occur (loss of central vision), usually in males, who may be young.
6. *Does he or she suffer from increasing headaches, giddiness, nausea, spontaneous vomiting?* Consider intracranial space-occupying lesions.
7. *Is the patient atopic?* Keratoconus (abnormal curvature of the cornea) may present with gradual visual distortion, usually in patients under 25. Keratoconus may be associated with atopy and Down's syndrome.

Eye examination

External

Normal, unless a dense cataract leads to a white pupil.

Visual acuity

Variable. Test for both reading and distance – with glasses or a pinhole if glasses are not available. If distance vision improves with a pinhole, the patient probably requires new glasses. Most of those in the 40–50 age group who have difficulty reading will require reading glasses. Macular disease (usually macular degeneration) makes vision worse with a pinhole.

Fields

Central loss occurs in advanced macular degeneration. Bitemporal field loss may occur in anterior cranial fossa tumours (compression of chiasm).

Pupils

Look at the red reflex (p. 6) as this may easily identify cataract. If an afferent pupil defect (p. 3) is present, this is due to anterior visual pathway pathology (gross retinal lesion or compressive lesion on optic nerve, for example). Cataract does not give rise to an afferent pupil defect.

Fundi

The fundus is difficult to visualize in the presence of cataract. ARM may be subtle and seen as a granular pigment scatter at the macula (the retina temporal to the disc) or may be obvious as marked pigmentation or scarring. Retinal haemorrhages may indicate diabetes or hypertension, both of which may lead to bilateral visual loss.

Disc

Suspect glaucoma if discs are cupped and a compressive lesion if optic disc pallor is present.

Disc cupping describes the excavated appearance of the disc in advanced glaucoma.

General examination

1. BP.
2. Urinalysis for diabetes.
3. If disc pallor or visual field loss are present, look for other signs of a space-occupying lesion.
4. If the patient is unkempt with a history suggestive of poor diet, heavy smoking and alcohol intake, suspect toxic or nutritional amblyopia (bilateral loss of central field).

Management

No management is required other than referring the patient, as below.

Referral

Cataract and ARM should be referred to a routine ophthalmology outpatient clinic.

If new glasses are required, direct the patient to an optician.

Any other positive eye findings, such as disc pallor, field loss and retinal haemorrhages should be discussed with the ophthalmologist within 24 hours and referred for assessment as advised (usually within 48 hours).

Follow-up

Ophthalmology outpatient department only.

Transient loss of vision

Features

Unilateral transient loss of vision lasting from a few seconds to minutes is usually caused by retinal ischaemia. The whole visual field or just the upper or lower part may be affected (Fig. 1.5, p. 8).
Bilateral transient loss is usually secondary to cerebral ischaemia.

Pain is not usually a feature, but headache may occur in carotid insufficiency, migraine and temporal arteritis.

Main causes

1. Platelet or cholesterol emboli in the retinal circulation, thrown off from atherosclerotic carotid arteries.
2. Atrial fibrillation, causing emboli.
3. Vertebrobasilar or gross carotid insufficiency leads to bilateral simultaneous transient loss.
4. Temporal arteritis.

5. Migraine.
6. Papilloedema.

Eye examination

External

Feel the temporal arteries. If solid, non-pulsatile or tender in a patient over 60 years, suspect temporal arteritis (see p. 72).

Visual acuity

Document this in each eye, with glasses if worn or with a pinhole.

Fields

Assess for any gross field defect in each quadrant of each eye (pp. 7–9).

Pupils

These are usually normal.

Fundi

Look for emboli, which appear as white specks within the retinal arterioles, either adjacent to the disc or more peripherally. Swelling of both optic discs occurs in the presence of raised intracranial pressure and should be regarded as papilloedema until proved otherwise. Papilloedema may rarely lead to unilateral disc swelling only.

General examination

1. Listen to the carotid arteries (in the angle of the jaw) for bruits. Emboli causing transient visual loss usually arise from the carotid bifurcation.
2. Listen for heart murmurs and check the pulse for atrial fibrillation.
3. Look for long tract signs (ataxia) or cranial nerve signs (sixth-nerve palsy – see p. 103 and Fig. 3.3(b), p. 99), indicating raised intracranial pressure if disc swelling is present.

Management

1. Consider temporal arteritis. See p. 72 for features and management.
2. BP. Treat if required.
3. Start on aspirin 75 mg p.o. o.d. if emboli, heart murmurs or carotid bruits are present and there are no contraindications to aspirin.
4. Papilloedema – see referral below.

Referral and follow-up

- Papilloedema – discuss with and refer immediately to the neurosurgeons.
- If the ESR is raised or there are any other features of temporal arteritis, treat (p. 72) and refer immediately to the ophthalmologist as there is a high risk of permanent blindness.
- If the ESR is normal, but a heart murmur, carotid bruit or atrial fibrillation is present, discuss with the physicians as the patient requires a cardiovascular work-up. The physicians will refer to the ophthalmologist if required.

- If emboli are visible on fundoscopy or the patient is a known arteriopath treat as in (3) above and refer to the physicians as an outpatient (early appointment).
- If you can find no cause, discuss with the ophthalmologist immediately and arrange an assessment within 24 hours.

Flashes, floaters and 'cobwebs'

Features

Flashes or sparks of light (photopsia) are seen in response to mechanical traction on the retina and are typical in posterior vitreous detachment (Fig. 3.1) where the vitreous gel peels away from the retinal surface. A migrainous visual aura usually consists of a zigzag line of light which flickers and moves across the visual field rather than isolated flashes.

Floaters are opacities within the vitreous gel which sway in front of the patient's field of vision with eye movements. These occur as a result of posterior vitreous detachment, haemorrhage within the vitreous (diabetics or following trauma), or may be long-standing, particularly in myopes (short-sighted patients) in whom these are more visible.

'*Cobwebs*' or '*hairs*' are floaters, but this is a characteristic description by patients, who describe trying to wipe away a cobweb or thread which appears to hang in front of their face.

Eye examination

Visual acuity

Document this for each eye with glasses if worn, or with a pinhole.

Fields

Check the fields (pp. 7–9) for any gross defect which may indicate retinal detachment.

Fundi

Look for evidence of retinal detachment (p. 79) or vitreous opacities, including haemorrhage (p. 78).

Management

In all cases the pupil requires to be dilated and a detailed examination of the retina made. This can only be adequately undertaken by the ophthalmologist.

Referral

All cases that are not typically migraine-related (usually a long history of similar symptoms) should be referred to the ophthalmologist within 24 hours.

Follow-up

Ophthalmologist only.

Double vision (diplopia)

Features

Diplopia is often worse in a particular direction of gaze, and may be vertical (one object above the other), horizontal or a mixture of the two (Fig. 3.2).

The patient may tilt the head or chin to overcome the problem.

Painful diplopia – main causes

1. *Trauma.*
2. *Compressive lesion* affecting the third, fourth or sixth nerves (usually aneurysm) or mass behind the eye.
3. *Temporal arteritis* (may be painless).
4. *Diabetes* (may also be painless).

Painless diplopia – main causes

1. *Hypertension and diabetes* leading to ischaemia of the nerve supply to the extraocular muscles in the elderly (not invariably painless).

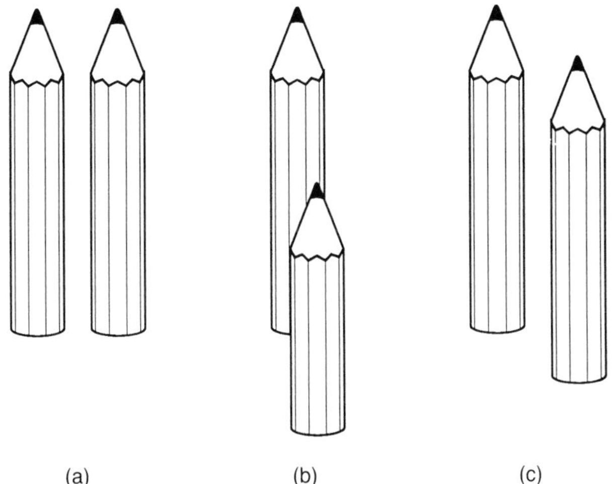

Fig. 3.2. Double vision (diplopia). (a) Horizontal diplopia; (b) vertical diplopia; (c) mixed horizontal and vertical diplopia.

2. *Dysthyroid eye disease*, resulting in mechanical restriction of extraocular muscles, usually in middle-aged women (pain/discomfort common in acute cases, p. 47).
3. *Demyelinating disease*, particularly in the young.
4. *Breakdown of childhood squint* – ask if the patient has previously had surgery or treatment for squint.
5. *Myasthenia gravis* – this is often associated with ptosis (drooping eyelid) at the end of the day.

Relevant questions

1. *Is it painful?*
   This is crucial, as a painful third-nerve palsy may indicate aneurysmal compression and is a neurosurgical emergency.
2. *Is the double vision horizontal, vertical or a mixture of both?*
   Horizontal diplopia usually signifies sixth-nerve palsy; vertical or skewed diplopia may be due to third- or fourth-nerve palsy, dysthyroid disease, mass behind the eye or blow-out fracture (this occurs when the orbital contents are forced through a fracture in the inferior orbit; Fig. 3.3a, p. 99).
3. *Is the patient a known hypertensive or diabetic?*
   Diabetic third-nerve palsy may be painful and impossible to distinguish clinically from an aneurysm.
4. *Was the onset sudden and painless?*
   This is usually secondary to an acute ischaemic episode.
5. *Is there evidence of temporal arteritis?*
   Headache, myalgia, weight loss, tender or solid temporal arteries, jaw claudication (see p. 72).

6. *Is there a history of trauma?*
Blunt injury to the orbit may lead to a blow-out fracture with double vision in upgaze.
7. *Is there a history of thyroid disease?*
Double vision on attempted upgaze is the most common manifestation (p. 47).

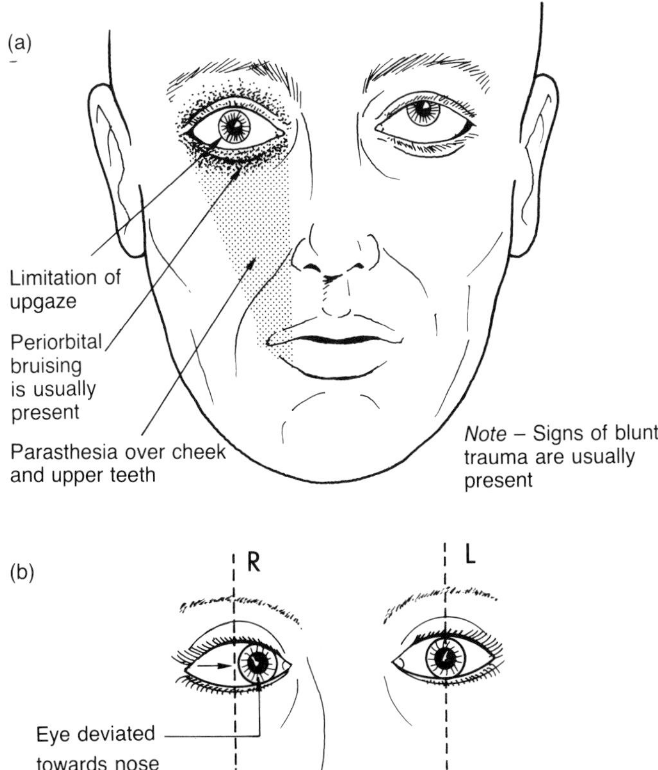

The eye may be able to cross the midline in a partial sixth-nerve palsy

Fig. 3.3. (a) Blow-out fracture; (b) sixth-nerve palsy; R, right lateral rectus palsy–patient looking straight ahead; L, failure of abduction, left lateral rectus palsy–patient looking left.

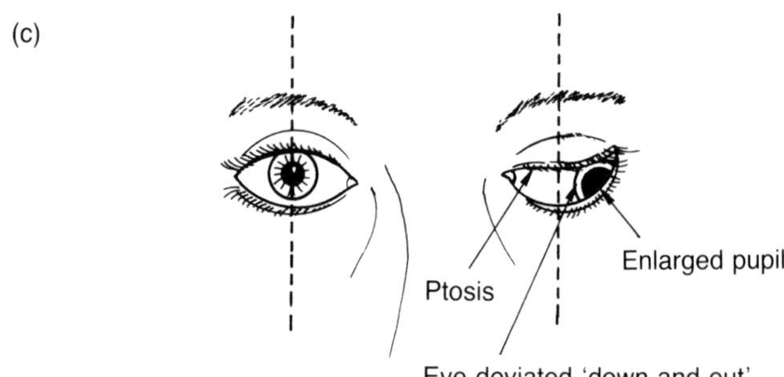

Sudden-onset painful third-nerve palsy is a neurosurgical emergency

Beware
1 Pupil may be spared (i.e. appears normal)
2 Ptosis may be absent
3 Partial third-nerve palsy may affect only one extraocular muscle

Fig. 3.3. (c) Third-nerve palsy.

8. *Are there any other neurological symptoms?* Weakness, paraesthesia or previous blurring of vision at any time in the past may indicate demyelinating disease.
9. *Does the patient tire easily or do the eyelids droop, particularly at the end of the day?* Consider myasthenia gravis. This is rare, but is usually missed.
10. *Is the double vision only in one eye?* Cataract may lead to monocular diplopia.

Eye examination

External

Feel the temporal arteries for evidence of arteritis (p. 72). Ptosis is associated with a third nerve palsy. Check eye movements (p. 2 and below).

Prominent eyes which may be white or injected are associated with dysthyroid eye disease.

If related to trauma, feel the orbital rim. A fracture line may be evident with overlying tenderness. If a blow-out fracture is suspected, touch the cheek with a piece of cotton wool lightly on each side for comparison. Numbness indicates infraorbital nerve involvement (see Trauma, p. 116).

Eye movements

Limitation of lateral gaze with horizontal diplopia is indicative of sixth-nerve palsy (Fig. 3.3b).

Limitation of virtually all movements with the exception of lateral gaze indicates third-nerve palsy if of acute onset. There may be an associated ptosis. This pattern (without ptosis) may be mimicked by restrictive thyroid orbital disease, and may be associated with bilateral red eyes. Limitation of upgaze with an increase in diplopia is associated with blow-out fracture and dysthyroid eye disease.

Visual acuity

Usually normal, but may be reduced in dysthyroid disease due to corneal exposure if eyes are very prominent, or compression of the optic nerve by increased orbital contents.

Fields

A field defect is rarely present.

Pupils

An enlarged pupil in the presence of a painful third-

nerve palsy indicates an aneurysm until proved otherwise (Fig. 3.3c). This is a neurosurgical emergency. Although a normal pupil is typical in diabetic or hypertensive nerve palsies, it can also occur in the presence of an aneurysm.

Cornea

Check sensation by rolling a small fragment of tissue to a soft point, then touching the corneal surface from the side so that the patient does not see the tissue approaching. Compare sensation in both eyes. Loss of sensation, particularly in association with an ipsilateral sixth-nerve palsy and hearing defect, suggests an acoustic neuroma.

Fundi

Usually normal. Diabetic patients may have retinopathy. Swollen optic discs signify papilloedema until proved otherwise and may also occur in temporal arteritis. Remember, however, that in papilloedema visual acuity is frequently normal, whereas in disc swelling, secondary to temporal arteritis, vision is profoundly reduced.

General examination

1. Examine for other injuries if trauma-related.
2. Blood pressure.
3. Urinalysis for diabetes.
4. Full cranial nerve examination.
5. ESR.

Management and referral

Painful third-nerve palsy with pupil involvement

Transfer the patient immediately by ambulance (not by car) to the neurosurgeons, and inform them of the patient's imminent arrival. Patients may die en route from aneurysmal rupture.

Third-nerve palsy with pupil sparing

Admit the patient under the neurosurgeon for observation. Pupil involvement may occur later. Pupil sparing, that is, a normal pupil in the presence of a third-nerve palsy, may occur in the presence of an aneurysm.

Sixth-nerve palsy

If associated with diabetes, hypertension or atherosclerotic disease, with absence of other neurological signs, arrange follow-up in 5–7 days after discussing with the ophthalmologist.

If corneal sensation or hearing is reduced, refer to the neurosurgeons within 24 hours.

Treat hypertension and discuss with physicians if the patient is a newly diagnosed diabetic.

Advise patient to reattend immediately if any new features develop.

Temporal arteritis (p. 72) may present as a sixth-nerve palsy (and rarely as a third-nerve palsy).

Traumatic

Traumatic cases of diplopia should be discussed with the ophthalmologist and seen urgently to exclude other ocular trauma. X-ray the orbits and paranasal sinuses and look for a blow-out fracture (opacity in the maxillary sinus, Plate 14), air in the orbit or blood in the sinuses. Treat prophylactically with systemic broad spectrum antibiotics (Magnapen 500 mg q.d.s. p.o. in adults) if there is evidence of a blow-out fracture or an open wound is present. Check tetanus status and treat if required.

Children complaining of double vision

All children should be urgently seen by an ophthalmologist, with the exception of a painful third-nerve palsy, which must be transferred urgently to the neurosurgeons as above.

Association with previous neurological deficits

This suggests demyelinating disease and should be referred to the neurologists within 48 hours.

Dysthyroid eye disease and proptosis

If associated with pain, reduced visual acuity or afferent pupil defect (p. 6), discuss with ophthalmologist immediately. Long-standing or intermittent diplopia is common, and should be routinely referred to the ophthalmology outpatient department.

Other cases

Those cases not falling into the above categories may have diplopia as a result of cataract (monocular diplopia), myasthenia (often worse at the end of the day), breakdown of long-standing ocular imbalance or previous surgery (after retinal detachment repair).

All should have an early ophthalmology outpatient appointment arranged.

Follow-up

Ophthalmology, neurology or neurosurgery outpatient department only.

Pitfall

Failure to treat a third-nerve palsy with pupil involvement as a neurosurgical emergency. These patients must be sent by ambulance to the neurosurgeons and may die en route.

4

Painful eye

This is a common complaint and is usually related to ocular trauma or inflammation.

Ascertain first:
Is the eye red? Go to p. 11
Is there a history of trauma? Go to p. 116
Is vision reduced? Go to p. 63
Is there double vision? Go to p. 96.

Painful eye, normal appearance, normal vision

Pain in or around a normal-looking eye is common, and frequently no cause can be identified.

Consider:
1. Temporal arteritis – if elderly p. 72.
2. Sinusitis – particularly if there is a past history p. 109.
3. Neuralgia – this may follow ophthalmic shingles p. 113.
4. Migraine – often associated with a strong family history p. 110.
5. Diabetes – non-specific pain which may occur with sixth-, third- or fourth-nerve palsy p. 97.
6. Optic neuritis – vision may be normal, but an afferent pupil defect is usually present p. 76.

Relevant questions

1. *Is temporal arteritis a possibility?*
   Consider this in the over-50s (usually over-70s) if

associated with malaise, weight loss, jaw pain with eating (claudication), shoulder girdle pain and scalp tenderness (p. 72).

2. *Is the pain in the eye itself, or surrounding the eye?* Patients often describe periocular pain as eye pain. Pain may be referred from the temporomandibular joint, ear or sinuses.
3. *Has there been a recent history of a cold or sinusitis?* Sinusitis may be recurrent and leads to a dull periocular pain.
4. *Does the patient have headaches or a past history of migraine?*
   There is often a strong family history.
5. *Is there a history of ophthalmic shingles?*
   Neuralgic pain following shingles may be persistent and severe long after the skin lesions have resolved.
6. *Is the patient diabetic, hypertensive or a smoker?*
   All may lead to ocular ischaemia and periocular pain, which is dull and persistent.
7. *Is the patient wearing old glasses, or having difficulty and pain when reading?*
   Incorrect glasses, or the need for spectacles, particularly in middle-aged patients who experience difficulty with reading, are a common cause of visual discomfort.

Eye examination

External

Erythema or fullness of the periocular tissues (Plate 1) occurs in periorbital or orbital cellulitis which may be sufficiently subtle to be missed unless specifically looked for (p. 150). Feel the temporal arteries – if tender, non-pulsatile or nodular, consider temporal arteritis (p. 72). Look for scars on the face and scalp from old ophthalmic shingles (herpes zoster ophthalmicus, HZO, p. 156) or trauma.

Lids

Feel the lid margins for cysts or styes. These are often less visible in dark-skinned individuals, and may be acutely tender.

Visual acuity

Document this for each eye individually, with glasses if worn, and with a pinhole if the patient has not brought glasses.

Pupils

An afferent pupil defect (p. 3) may occur in optic neuritis and compressive lesions such as a mucocoele pressing on the optic nerve. If there is a pupil defect, ensure that there is no other cranial nerve palsy (p. 102). If one pupil is larger, consider a third-nerve palsy (p. 103).

Eye movements

Double vision may occur via a nerve palsy of the extraocular muscles (p. 97), orbital restriction secondary to thyroid eye disease (p. 47) or orbital mass.

Cornea

Stain the cornea with dilute fluorescein (make sure contact lenses are removed first), and look for an abrasion (p. 16) or a foreign body (p. 18, plates 4 and 5) as the eye may appear normal despite these conditions in the early stages.

Fundus

There are usually no fundal findings in the absence of trauma or previous surgery; however, haemorrhages may be visible in diabetics and those with ocular ischaemia.

Temporal arteritis

Features and management

This is fully discussed on p. 72.

Sinusitis

Features

There is often a recurrent history of sinusitis, recent upper respiratory infection, production of mucus, headache or fever. Pain may be acute or chronic, often relapsing.

Associations

Smoking.

Management

1. Ensure that visual acuity, pupils and eye movements are normal.

2. Tap with your index finger over the frontal and maxillary sinuses. Tenderness supports the diagnosis.
3. X-ray the paranasal and periorbital sinuses if the diagnosis is in doubt.
4. Start oral antibiotics. Magnapen 500 mg q.d.s. (ampicillin 250 mg and flucloxacillin 250 mg combination tablet) p.o. for 10 days is usually effective.

Referral

- Discuss with the ophthalmologist urgently if there is double vision or a pupil defect.
- Refer to the ear, nose and throat department if there are frequent recurrences of sinusitis.
- No referral is required if there are no ocular findings, and symptoms settle on the above treatment.

Follow-up

- No follow-up is required if symptoms settle. However, advise the patient to reattend immediately should visual symptoms develop or if symptoms do not settle on treatment within 72 hours.
- If the patient is referred as above, follow-up will be arranged by the relevant specialist.

Migraine

Features

The history may be classical with headache, nausea, vomiting and visual aura, classically zigzag lights which move progressively across the visual field (fortification spectra). Pain is usually acute, throbbing and unilateral, and may last for days (usually up to a maximum of 48 hours). Variants include sudden, transient loss of all or part of the visual field, which may very rarely become permanent. Headache may not occur. Vision is usually normal between episodes, but rarely, loss can occur due to retinal arteriolar spasm (see CRAO, p. 69) or occipital damage. Visual fields are usually normal; however, many and varied defects can occur.

Associations

Oral contraceptive pill, chocolate, cheese, stress. Often strong family history.

Management

1. Check blood pressure.
2. Document visual acuities and field to confrontation.
3. If the patient is over 50, check the erythrocyte sedimentation rate (ESR), look for signs and symptoms of temporal arteritis and treat appropriately if you suspect this (p. 72).
4. Simple analgesia initially, e.g. paracetamol 1 g p.o. q.d.s. Advise rest in a quiet dark room.
5. Antiemetics if required. Metoclopromide (Maxolon) 10 mg p.o./i.m. or prochlorperazine (Stemetil) 5.0 mg p.o. or 12.5 mg i.m. Give i.m. doses if vomiting is a feature rather than simply nausea.
6. Sumatriptan (Imigran) subcutaneously or orally may be rapidly effective in true migraine.
7. Fundus examination – usually normal, but look for disc swelling and vitreous haemorrhage which may be associated with subarachnoid haemorrhage.

8. If episodes are frequent, treat prophylactically (best done by the GP).

Referral

- Reduced visual acuity or field loss – discuss with ophthalmologist immediately. Retinal arteriolar spasm can occur (p. 69). See Pitfall, below.
- If the history is typical or the patient has a history of migraines, and there are no ocular findings, reassure the patient, and refer to the GP for prophylaxis if episodes are frequent.
- If attending GP with frequent migraines, treat prophylactically, and refer to neurologist if symptoms do not improve.
- If there is no previous history and the patient is over 30, refer to neurology outpatient department (soon) as this may be secondary to other pathology (reactive migraine).

Follow-up

Only routine migraine control and assessment by the patient's GP is required in typical cases. If referred to neurology, they will arrange follow-up.

Pitfall

Occipital pain – consider subarachnoid haemorrhage if pain is severe and of sudden onset. Look for a field defect (not always present). Discuss with neurosurgeons immediately as a small bleed may precede a large one.

See Transient loss of vision, p. 92.

Neuralgia

Features

Dull or lancinating pain which may be chronic or intermittent. Consider cluster headache, which usually affects males and causes excruciating periorbital pain and rhinorrhoea for several hours per day. The eye may be red and waters.

Associations

Previous history of ophthalmic shingles, diabetes, local trauma, migraine.

Management

1. Consider temporal arteritis, and check ESR in a patient over 50, particularly if there are other clinical signs. This is fully discussed on p. 72.
2. Check blood pressure and urinalysis. Treat appropriately.
3. Simple analgesia. The patient frequently has not tried any simple analgesia such as paracetamol.
4. If related to ophthalmic shingles (HZO), look for uveitis (inflammation within the eye, p. 23) Intraocular pressure may be elevated.
5. Variable success occurs with:
   (a) Transcutaneous nerve stimulation (TENS) – see Referral below.
   (b) Amitriptyline 25 mg o.d. p.o. starting dose (beware urinary retention, cardiotoxic).
   (c) Carbamazepine (Tegretol) 100 mg nocte p.o. (narrow therapeutic range).
   (d) Acupuncture.

Referral

- Previous HZO – discuss with ophthalmologist.
- Physiotherapist for TENS and acupuncture.
- If persistent and severe, refer to neurologist (out-patient department, soon) or pain clinic if one is available. Obtain advice from physicians prior to starting amitriptyline or carbamazepine.

Follow-up

If referral to another specialist is made as above, they will arrange follow-up and refer back to you if required. In the absence of any findings on examination, no routine follow-up is required, but advise the patient to return immediately should any new signs or symptoms occur (field defect, diplopia, any neurological changes).

Diabetic patient

Features

Pain may be acute or chronic and mimic that of herpetic neuralgia.

Management

1. Check blood pressure and urine.
2. Document the visual acuity, with glasses if these are worn, or with a pinhole.
3. Check eye movements and ask the patient if he or she sees double in any position (diplopia), as

diabetic neuropathy may be painful, and can affect the third, fourth or sixth nerves (pp. 98 and 103).

4. Look for diabetic retinopathy (haemorrhages, exudates, engorged vessels), and document this.
5. Try simple analgesia, e.g. paracetamol 1 g p.o. qds. The neuralgia usually resolves spontaneously over a few days.

Referral

If there are any ocular findings, discuss with ophthalmologist immediately.

Persistent pain should be referred to the physicians (outpatient department, soon) for diabetic assessment.

New diabetics and hypertensives should be treated initially by the primary care team, and referred to the physicians if appropriate.

Follow-up

Those with retinopathy will be followed-up by the ophthalmologist or diabetic team, who will refer back to the GP as appropriate.

Pitfall

Failure to recognize and refer diabetic retinopathy. Untreated proliferative disease may rapidly lead to permanent visual disability and subsequent litigation.

5

Trauma

Chemical injury see p. 38
Corneal abrasion see p. 16
Corneal foreign body see p. 18

1. Blunt injury see below
2. Sharp injury p. 128.

Blunt injury (Fig. 5.1)

1. Suspected globe rupture or penetrating injury p. 121.
2. Orbital haematoma – with and without view of eye p. 122.
3. Double vision (suspected blow-out fracture) p. 124. See Fig. 3.3a, p. 99.
4. Hyphaema p. 126. See Fig. 5.1, p. 117 and Plate 11.

Usual cause

1. Assault – usually a fist punch.
2. Sporting injuries – squash ball, football or shuttlecock injury and contact sport.

Relevant questions

1. *Obtain and document an accurate history.*
   This is particularly important in trauma. Document the time of injury, and the exact cause. Injuries from a squash ball or shuttlecock can be

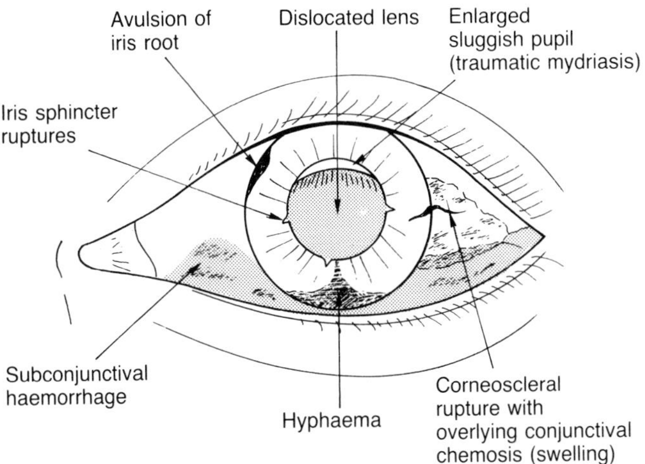

Fig. 5.1. Blunt trauma – features.

particularly severe, as they 'fit' neatly into the eye socket. Children frequently do not tell the truth concerning mode of injury as they may fear parental punishment.

2. *Was the patient knocked out?*
   You will need to treat as a head-injury case in addition to ocular injury.
3. *Is vision reduced?*
   This may be secondary to a corneal abrasion (p. 16, Plates 4 and 5) or internal ocular bleeding. A hyphaema is a blood level seen in the front of the eye (Fig. 5.1, Plate 11), obscuring the lower portion of the iris. Rarely, it may be sufficiently severe to obscure most or all of the iris. Retinal bruising and detachment may occur.
4. *Does the patient see double?*
   Orbital contents may be forced through the thin lower orbital floor into the maxillary sinus – a

blow-out fracture (Plate 14). This leads to tethering of the eye in attempted upgaze and vertical diplopia (i.e. one image vertically above the other; see Figs 3.2, p. 97 and 3.3, p. 99).

Examination

Ensure there are no other severe non-ocular injuries that require urgent management.

External

Periorbital bruising may be so severe that the eye cannot be opened (Plate 1). Feel the orbital rim for tenderness or bony fractures. Carefully examine wounds on the lids or upper cheek – these may be sufficiently deep to involve the globe. Crepitus indicates a fracture of the medial wall of the orbit.

Lids

Look for lacerations in the lid, including the lid margin, as these may indicate underlying ocular damage. Attempt to prise open the lids gently if swollen or haemorrhagic to obtain a view of the globe.

External globe

If the globe looks distorted, or it is difficult to recognize normal features, it may be ruptured. *Do not attempt any further examination.* Subconjunctival haemorrhage is common (Plate 3), and appears as a solid red discoloration of the normal white of the eye. There may be associated oedema of the conjunctiva, which appears as a water-logged membrane, usually in the lower fornix (covering the lower part of the globe).

Visual acuity

It is essential to document this *in each eye individually*, using a pinhole if the patient usually wears glasses. Reduced vision is commonly associated with corneal abrasions (p. 16), hyphaema and retinal bruising.

Eye movements

These are frequently restricted as a result of orbital oedema. Restricted upgaze with double vision is typical of a blow-out fracture (see Fig. 3.3a, p. 99).

Cornea

Stain the cornea with fluorescein and look for an abrasion under a blue light (p. 16; Plate 4). Full-thickness corneal and scleral lacerations may occur in blunt trauma.

Iris and pupil

A hyphaema (blood level) may obscure the lower part of the iris, and indicates significant ocular injury (Plate 10). Pupil distortion may indicate penetrating injury. The pupil may be dilated and sluggish as a result of trauma (traumatic mydriasis). However, in the presence of a tight periorbital haematoma (Plate 1), an afferent pupil defect indicates a compromised optic nerve as a result of raised orbital pressure, which requires urgent decompression (see Lateral canthotomy, p. 124).

Lens

An opaque lens may indicate an associated penetrating injury. Severe injury may dislocate the lens.

Fundus

Retinal pallor and haemorrhages indicate retinal 'bruising' (commotio retinae). This may lead to retinal detachment, which appears as a grey floating 'curtain' on fundoscopy (p. 79). This may be apparent at initial presentation, frequently with an associated vitreous haemorrhage (p. 78).

All blunt ocular injuries should be reviewed by an ophthalmologist:

- *Immediately* — Globe rupture, globe penetration, pupil defect with a dense periorbital haematoma, child with hyphaema or visual loss.
- *Within 24 hours (discuss immediately)* — Reduced visual acuity, hyphaema in an adult, lid-margin lacerations, retinal haemorrhages, blow-out fracture, children with no hyphaema and no visual loss.
- *Within 48 hours* — Normal eye, but periorbital bruising.

Suspected globe rupture or penetrating injury

Features

Distorted globe or pupil, swollen haemorrhagic conjunctiva, full-thickness lid lacerations.

Management

1. Cover eye with eye shield. Do not put any pressure on the globe at all or you may cause expulsion of intraocular contents.
2. Document the visual acuity in both eyes – record the fact that you have attempted to document vision, even if unsuccessful.
3. Do not instil any drops.
4. Cover with systemic antibiotics, e.g. cefuroxime 1.5 g i.v.
5. Check tetanus status and treat appropriately.
6. X-ray the orbit and paranasal sinuses, and look for fluid levels, air or prolapsed tissue (Plate 14).
7. Keep patient fasted until seen by ophthalmologist.

Referral

Ophthalmologist immediately.

Follow-up

Ophthalmologist only.

Orbital haematoma with no view of eye

Features

A tense, swollen periorbital haematoma (Plate 1) may rarely cause optic nerve compression.

Management

1. Gently place an ice pack over the lids to try and reduce swelling.
2. If associated with an open skin wound, check tetanus status and treat appropriately.
3. X-ray the orbit and paranasal sinuses, and look for fluid levels, air or prolapsed orbital tissue into maxillary sinus (blow-out fracture, p. 124 Plate 14 and Fig. 3.3a, p. 99).

Referral

Discuss with ophthalmologist immediately.

Follow-up

Ophthalmologist only.

Orbital haematoma with a view of the eye

Features

The eye may be spared or severely injured. Retinal damage may occur in the absence of any surface damage.

Management

1. Document visual acuity.
2. Attempt to identify whether the globe is intact. The cornea should be visible, as should the pupil, unless there is an associated hyphaema.
3. Check pupil for afferent defect (rare in these cases, p. 3). Pupil may be enlarged and sluggish as a result of sphincter damage.
4. Look for a hyphaema (Plate 11) and treat appropriately (p. 126).
5. Attempt to visualize fundus, even if only optic disc is seen. Document this.
6. Stain the cornea with fluorescein and treat any associated corneal abrasion (p. 16, Plate 4).
7. If there is an open skin wound, check tetanus status and treat appropriately.
8. X-ray orbit and paranasal sinuses, and look for sinus opacities (Plate 14).
9. Document presence or absence of infraorbital nerve paraesthesia, characterized by numbness over cheek and upper teeth (see Fig. 3.3a, p. 99), double vision in any direction of gaze (particularly vertical diplopia when attempting to look up; Figs 3.2, p. 97 and 3.3a). These are signs of a blow-out fracture (see below).
10. Place an ice pack on the haematoma unless there is evidence of globe rupture or penetration.

Referral

Suspected globe rupture – refer immediately to the ophthalmologist.
Afferent pupil defect – refer immediately to the ophthalmologist if associated with a tight haematoma, as this indicates compression of the optic

nerve. A sluggish pupil may simply be traumatic mydriasis, but discuss any pupil abnormality with the ophthalmologist. If a long delay is anticipated before the patient is seen by the ophthalmologist, and you suspect optic nerve compression, sight may be saved by a lateral canthotomy, as follows:

Lateral canthotomy

1. Clamp up to 1 cm of the outer canthus (junction between the upper and lower lids) with a pair of artery forceps for 30 seconds.
2. Cut along the line of crushed tissue with scissors. This can usually be done without local anaesthetic, which will only further increase tissue volume.

Globe intact and normal visual acuity – refer to ophthalmologist within 24 hours.

Orbital bruising and double vision – suspected 'blow-out' fracture

Features

Double vision in upgaze and paraesthesia along the course of the infraorbital nerve (cheek, upper lip and upper teeth) indicates a blow-out fracture, where orbital contents are forced through the lower orbital plate into the maxillary sinus (Plate 14 and Fig. 3.3a, p. 99).

Management

1. Treat as for orbital haematoma with a view of the eye, as above.

2. Cover with systemic antibiotics, e.g. Magnapen 500 mg p.o. q.d.s.
3. Check tetanus status and treat as required if an open skin wound is present.

Referral

Ophthalmologist within 24 hours.

Follow-up

Ophthalmologist only.

Subconjunctival haemorrhage

Features

Solid red discoloration of the conjunctiva (Plate 3). Frequently sharply demarcated from normal white regions.

Management and referral

All traumatic subconjunctival haemorrhages should be discussed with the ophthalmologist. If globe looks intact, and visual acuity and pupils are normal, refer within 24 hours. If any other abnormalities, refer immediately, as a subconjunctival haemorrhage may overly a globe rupture.

Follow-up

Ophthalmologist only.

Hyphaema

Features

Blood level seen in the anterior chamber of the eye (Plate 11). May be barely visible or may fill the eye.

Management

1. Document visual acuity.
2. Stain the cornea, look for an abrasion (Plates 4 and 5), and if present treat appropriately (p. 16).
3. Ensure globe is intact. A soft distorted eye indicates globe rupture, and is rare.
4. Strict bed rest reduces the risk of a rebleed, which is most likely to occur 3–5 days following injury. A rebleed is usually more severe than the initial bleed and can lead to loss of the eye.
5. Do not dilate the pupil. Leave this to the ophthalmologist.
6. Predsol drops t.d.s. reduce posttraumatic uveitis.

Referral

Children – admit under the ophthalmologists.
Hyphaemas greater than one-third corneal diameter – admit under ophthalmologists.
Small hyphaemas – Discuss with ophthalmologist. If the patient is a sensible adult, advise strict bed rest and arrange ophthalmological review within 24 hours.

Follow-up

Ophthalmologist only.

Pitfall

Failure to advise patient strongly of necessity of absolute bed rest, and to document this advice, as a rebleed can lead to loss of the eye.

Lid lacerations

Features

May be full-thickness and involve the globe. Medial lacerations may damage the lacrimal apparatus. Animal bites and road traffic accident injuries may avulse whole portions of the lid(s).

Management

1. Check for other associated ocular injuries and treat appropriately.
2. Ascertain wound depth. If full-thickness, the globe may also be involved.
3. If partial thickness and not through the lid margin, clean and repair with 6/0 silk or Vicryl or Prolene to the skin.
4. If full-thickness or involving lid margin or lacrimal puncta (approximately the medial quarter of lids), leave repair to the ophthalmologist.
5. Check tetanus status and treat appropriately.
6. Place loose, sterile dressing over wound.

Referral

If you suspect an underlying ocular rupture or penetration, refer immediately. Lid lacerations can otherwise be left for 24 hours before being seen by the ophthalmologist. Minor lacerations with no associated ocular injury can be repaired without any ophthalmological referral. Remove sutures after 6 days.

Follow-up

Six days for suture removal in uncomplicated cases. Ophthalmologist will review all others.

Sharp and penetrating injuries (Fig. 5.2)

Usual causes

1. *High-velocity particles* – usually metallic fragments from metal-on-metal impact, e.g. hammering on a nail or chisel, airgun injuries pp. 131, 133.

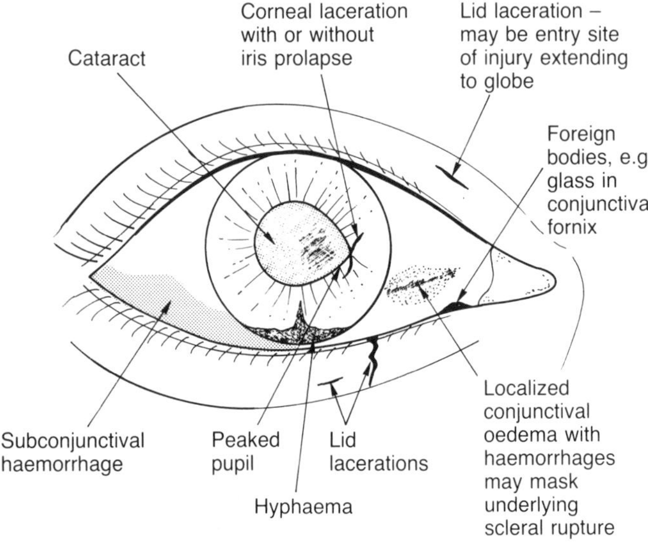

Fig. 5.2. Sharp injury – features.

2. *Thrown objects* – usually children with screwdrivers, scissors and knives p. 131.
3. *Gardening* – patient may bend down on to a spike of a shrub or supporting stick p. 131.
4. *Glass injuries* – usually following assault with a broken bottle or glass p. 131.

Accurately document the time and cause of injury. Children may not tell the truth if they fear punishment.

Relevant questions

1. *What exactly was the patient doing, and at what time was the injury? Was he or she wearing protective goggles?*
   Document answers to these questions carefully.
2. *Did the patient feel an impact, and if so, where?*
   Look carefully for a site of entry, which may be extremely small. High-velocity particles may travel through a considerable amount of tissue and still have sufficient energy to penetrate the globe.
3. *Is vision affected?*
   Lens opacity and vitreous haemorrhage may be present. Vision may be normal despite the presence of an intraocular foreign body.

Examination

External

Blood may obscure detailed examination, particularly in glass injuries associated with multiple lacerations. Do *not* attempt to clean or remove fragments near the eye or surrounding tissue – it is easy to cause even more injury.

Lids

Even small lid lacerations may be full-thickness and involve the globe. Look for small puncture wounds in the upper or lower lids (see Fig. 5.2, p. 128), and just below the eyebrow.

Visual acuity

Attempt to assess and document. Visual acuity is often reduced due to blood which may be either external or intraocular. Do not put pressure on lids to try and open them – this may lead to prolapse of intraocular tissue.

Conjunctiva

Subconjunctival haemorrhage may overlie the site of a penetrating injury, particularly if there is associated local oedema.

Cornea

Look for evidence of penetration (Plate 8). Stain with 2% fluorescein. This may demonstrate aqueous leakage in full-thickness injuries. Iris may prolapse through such a wound.

Lens

This may become opaque shortly (usually over an hour) after being punctured. Look at the red reflex

(p. 6). This may show corneal irregularities as well as lens and vitreous opacities.

Pupil

Pupil distortion (see Fig. 5.2, p. 128) is associated with penetrating injuries affecting the anterior part of the eye, but may appear normal with posterior penetrating injuries.

Fundus

Attempt to obtain a fundal view, but do not persevere if difficult. Blood frequently obscures the view.

X-ray

Orbit and paranasal sinuses (Plate 12). Even glass fragments are occasionally radio-opaque. Medicolegal difficulties may arise at a later date if this investigation is omitted.

Injuries due to thrown projectiles, glass, airgun pellets and gardening

Features

These are usually obvious. If you are in doubt as to whether penetration has occurred, treat as a penetrating injury.

Management

1. Document visual acuity if possible.
2. If you suspect globe rupture, cover with an eye

shield (do not touch the eye at all), do not instil any drops, and *do not attempt further examination*.

3. If the globe is intact, instil dilute fluorescein carefully and gently examine for corneal abrasions (p. 16 and Plate 4). Examine the folds of conjunctiva in the gutter between the eye and the lower lid by making the patient look up and gently pulling the lower lid down. Foreign body fragments may lie here. Gently remove with a cotton bud.
4. Foreign bodies not easily removed should be left for the ophthalmologist to remove.
5. Do not evert the upper lid if there is any possibility of a penetrating injury – you may expulse intraocular contents.
6. Cover with systemic antibiotics, e.g. cefuroxime 1.5 g i.v. if penetration suspected.
7. Check tetanus status and treat as appropriate.
8. X-ray the orbit and paranasal sinuses (Plates 12 and 14). A normal X-ray does not exclude an intraocular foreign body. Glass with a high lead content may show on X-ray.
9. Keep fasted until seen by ophthalmologist.

Referral

Immediately to the ophthalmologist.

Follow-up

Ophthalmologist only.

Pitfalls

See under Hammering, chiselling or similar, below.

Hammering, chiselling or similar

Features

Small, high-velocity metal fragments can penetrate the globe with little to find on examination and few, if any, symptoms. Puncture sites in the periorbital skin may indicate the entry site of a particle which has gone on to penetrate the globe. Small corneal puncture wound sites may be easily missed.

Management

1. Document visual acuity.
2. Treat any associated corneal abrasion (p. 16) and remove any superficial corneal foreign body. If a foreign body does not appear superficial, do not attempt to remove it.
3. If there is a skin laceration, check tetanus status and treat appropriately.
4. X-ray the orbit (Plate 12) – include lateral views.

Referral

All cases must be seen by the ophthalmologist if there is any doubt about the presence of an intraocular foreign body.
If penetration is obvious – refer immediately.
If there is doubt about penetration – discuss with ophthalmologist immediately. A cataract may develop quite rapidly following a penetrating injury, making subsequent fundus examination impossible by normal methods.
Children – refer immediately.

Follow-up

Ophthalmologist only.

Pitfalls

It is not uncommon for an intraocular foreign body to be missed, sometimes for months. The patient may present later with an acutely inflamed eye, or gradual loss of vision. Litigation may occur. A negative X-ray – even a negative computed tomography scan – does not rule out the possibility of an intraocular foreign body. If a superficial corneal foreign body is obvious, it is reasonable simply to remove and treat this (p. 18).

The majority of potential problems may be avoided by:

1. Accurately documenting the history.
2. Accurately documenting a thorough examination.
3. Taking an X-ray of the orbit.
4. Referring to the ophthalmologist if there is any doubt.

6 Contact lens-related

This is a frequent problem and usually related to:

1. Contact lens overwear – usually overnight p. 135.
2. Accidental instillation of contact lens cleaning fluid into eye p. 136.
3. Chronic irritation and lens intolerance p. 137.
4. Lost lenses – often after sporting trauma p. 139.
5. Corneal ulcers secondary to lens wear p. 27.

The patient usually gives an accurate history, and diagnosis is rarely a problem.

Contact lens overwear

Features

Acutely red eye, frequently bilateral, painful with a watery 'discharge'. This is common and usually occurs as a result of failing to remove contact lenses overnight.

Management

1. Confirm that contact lenses have been removed.
2. Instil a drop of topical anaesthetic to allow examination.
3. Stain the cornea with fluorescein. A diffuse pattern of staining is common centrally.
4. Look for a corneal ulcer and if present treat and refer appropriately (p. 27).
5. Instil a drop of homatropine 1% or cyclopentolate

1% (Mydrilate) to dilate the pupil and relieve painful ciliary muscle spasm if light is painful (photophobia). Advise patient to wear dark glasses for 1–2 days.
6. Instil chloramphenicol ointment 1%.
7. Patch the eye, or the worst eye if both eyes are involved, with a double pad (p. 17) for 24-hours.
8. Advise patient to leave out contact lenses during treatment.

Referral and follow-up

Not required unless a corneal ulcer is present, in which case refer to the ophthalmologist immediately (see p. 27).

Accidental instillation of lens-cleaning solution

Features

This is usually unilateral but may be bilateral. Acute pain with watery 'discharge'.

Management

1. Ensure contact lenses have been removed. If unable to open eyes, proceed to (2) first.
2. Instil a drop of topical anaesthetic to allow examination.
3. Remove the lenses if still *in situ* and irrigate using a free running drip set connected to a 1 litre bag of normal saline, with the patient lying down (p. 38). If the lenses have already been previously removed by the patient for over an hour, irrigation is unnecessary.

4. Stain with fluorescein. Diffuse punctate staining is usually present, indicating chemical damage. Look for a corneal ulcer and treat appropriately (p. 27).
5. Treat as an abrasion (p. 16) and patch the worst eye if bilateral.
6. In severe cases instil a drop of homatropine 1% or cyclopentolate 1% (Mydrilate) to relieve pain.
7. Discharge on chloramphenicol 1% ointment q.d.s. for 5 days.
8. Instruct patient to leave out contact lenses until they have been checked for foreign bodies by their optician, and not to reinsert them for a minimum of 1 week.

Referral and follow-up

Immediately to the ophthalmologist – corneal ulcer.
Review after 24 hours – severe bilateral punctate staining and, if not improving, discuss with the ophthalmologist.
Not required – mild unilateral or bilateral corneal staining.
Advise the patient to attend optician as in (8) above if appropriate.

Intolerance to contact lens wear

Features

This may occur even after several years of trouble-free contact lens wear and may be exacerbated by a change in the style of lens (e.g. hard to soft) or cleaning solution. May present as chronic ocular irritation.

Management

1. Remove contact lenses if *in situ*.
2. Evert the upper lid (Fig. 1.4, p. 7) by asking the patient to look down, and keep looking down. Place the wooden stick of a cotton bud horizontally across the mid-portion of the upper lid, grasp the eyelashes firmly and gently rotate the lid upwards over the stick. Remove the stick and hold the eyelid in position by holding the lashes. A red irregular undersurface usually indicates a chronic allergic response.
3. Stain the cornea with fluorescein. Punctate staining (multiple small dots) may be present if lenses are not adequately cleaned or do not fit correctly. Look for a corneal ulcer – this appears as a solid-staining area. Treat and refer appropriately (p. 27).
4. If corneal staining is present, and there is no evidence of corneal ulceration, discharge on chloramphenicol ointment 1% q.d.s. for 1 week.
5. If there is no corneal staining, but subtarsal (under upper lid) conjunctival injection is present, start on Alomide 0.1% drops q.d.s to both eyes. Lenses should not be inserted whilst on treatment.
6. Lenses should not be reinserted until the patient has been seen by their optician.

Referral and follow-up

Immediately to ophthalmologist – corneal ulcer.
Review within 24 hours – marked diffuse corneal staining and, if no improvement, refer to ophthalmologist within 24 hours.
Optician – mild or no corneal staining.

Lost contact lens

Features

This can occur spontaneously or more typically after sport. Soft lenses may cause few symptoms despite being folded under the upper lid.

Management

1. Ensure that the patient has not in fact removed the lens.
2. Instil a drop of topical anaesthetic.
3. Examine with a slitlamp if available, otherwise under a good light. Look in the lower conjunctival fornix (the gutter between the lower eyelid and the globe) by making the patient look up whilst you pull the lower lid down. Ask the patient to look left and right whilst looking up, and look for the lens in the folds of conjunctiva.
4. Evert the upper lid (see Fig. 1.4, p. 7) by asking the patient to look down, and keep looking down. Place the wooden stick of a cotton bud horizontally across the mid-portion of the upper lid, grasp the eyelashes firmly and gently rotate the lid upwards over the stick. Remove the stick and hold the eyelid in position by holding the lashes. Make the patient look left and right in downgaze. Place the cotton bud under the upper lid into the upper conjunctival fornix and sweep it once (this is uncomfortable).
5. If the lens is still not found, instil fluorescein and observe under a blue light. If the patient has soft lenses, advise him or her before instilling the drop that this will stain the lens. Fluorescein will highlight the lens.

6. Repeat steps (3) and (4).
7. If the lens is found, ensure that it is intact. If part is missing, search for this.
8. Discharge on chloramphenicol ointment 1% q.d.s. for 1 week, and advise the patient not to reinsert the lens for this period.
9. Patch the eye for 24 hours if an abrasion is present (p. 16).
10. Advise patient to have lenses examined by their optician for damage, prior to re-inserting.

Referral

Only required if lens is not found, or part is missing. In these cases, instil chloramphenicol ointment, pad the eye, and refer to the ophthalmologist within 24 hours.

Follow-up

Not required unless a severe corneal abrasion is present. If so, review in 24 hours.

Corneal ulcer following contact lens wear

This is most common in soft and disposable lens wearers and is fully discussed under Corneal ulcers, on p. 27.

7

Watering eye

If associated with:
Red eye see p. 11.
Trauma see p. 116.
Watering is a normal physiological response in most cases.

Chronic watering in an otherwise quiet eye

Features

Often worse outdoors and in the wind. Frequently nuisance value only rather than major problem and more common in old age. Children born with watering eyes as a result of an incompletely developed nasolacrimal system frequently resolve spontaneously within 1 year.

Main causes

Adult

1. **Senile entropion and ectropion of lower lid** – usually bilateral, but watering may be unilateral.
2. **Stenosis (narrowing) of lacrimal punctum** – usually bilateral, but watering may be unilateral.
3. **Blockage of nasolacrimal system** – usually unilateral. A mucocoele may be present (p. 163).
4. **Blepharitis** – invariably bilateral. Lid crusting and inflammation, with or without an associated red eye (p. 146).
5. **Dry eye** – watering secondary to corneal irritation – bilateral.

Child

1. **Failure of canalization of nasolacrimal duct.**
2. **Congenital glaucoma**. Extremely rare. The eyes may look larger than normal – 'beautiful big eyes'. Photophobic (painful to look at light)

Examination

1. The bottom lid may not be closely applied to the eye – ectropion (Fig. 7.1). A gutter thus forms, fills with tears and overflows. This is common in the elderly, and may occur after lower-lid trauma in all age groups.
2. The medial part of the lower lid may be slightly turned out (medial ectropion), leading to drying and closure (stenosis) of the lacrimal puntum (the small duct responsible for tear drainage, Fig. 7.1).
3. The lower lid may turn in (entropion) allowing eyelashes to abrade the cornea (trichiasis, see Fig.

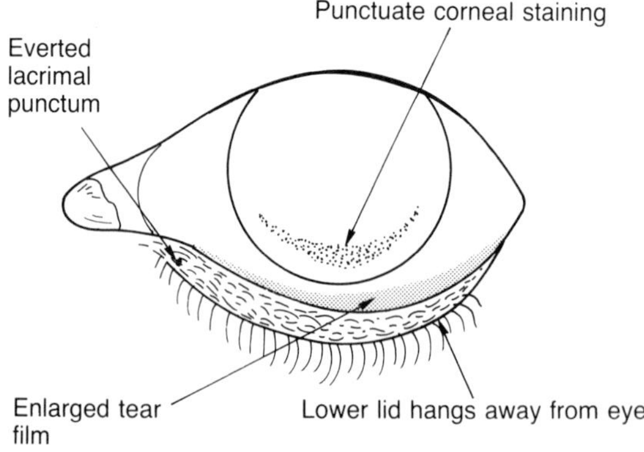

Fig. 7.1. Ectropion.

2.1a, p. 22). This produces chronic irritation and subsequent watering.

4. Feel for a palpable mass in the angle between the eye and nose – a mucocoele. Pressure may result in mucopus being expressed into the tear film.
5. Look for crusting of the lashes and erythema of the lid margin present with blepharitis (p. 46).
6. Stain the cornea with fluorescein and examine under a blue light on the slitlamp. Fine diffuse staining may indicate a dry eye. This is associated with secondary watering. If the tear film does not efficiently cover the whole of the cornea, dry patches may develop, despite the eye watering.

Management and referral – adult

- **Blepharitis** see p. 146.
- **Ectropion** see p. 158.
- **Entropion** see p. 157 and Fig. 2.1, p. 22.

- **Stenosis of lacrimal punctum**

No casualty/GP management.

Referral

Routine ophthalmology outpatient department.

- **Mucocoele (see p. 163)**

No casualty/GP management.

Referral

Routine ophthalmology outpatient department.

- **Dry eye**

Hypromellose 0.3% drops q.d.s. and Lacri-Lube ointment t.d.s. to the affected eye (usually bilateral).

Referral

Unnecessary unless corneal defects persist despite above treatment, in which case refer to the ophthalmology outpatient department routinely.

Management and referral – child

- **Failure of canalization of nasolacrimal duct**

Features

Chronic watering, often unilateral, having initially been bilateral, chronic conjunctivitis.

Management

1. Reassure parents – the condition usually resolves spontaneously by 12 months of age.
2. Keep the eye clean by gently washing away encrusted debris.
3. Massage to lacrimal sac. With forefinger, gently massage downwards from the corner of the eye halfway down the side of the nose 10 times, three times daily.

Referral

Ophthalmology outpatient department soon (non-urgent). If grossly infected, refer to ophthalmologist within 24 hours.

• **Suspected congenital glaucoma**

Features

Big eyes (typically described by relatives as having 'beautiful big eyes'), cloudy corneas, watering eyes, photophobia, parental concern with vision.

Referral

Ophthalmologist within 24 hours.

8 Lids

The most common complaints regarding the eyelids are:

1. Irritation, see below.
2. Infection, pp. 149–154.
3. Cysts and other lumps, p. 154.

Less common:

1. Entropion and ectropion, p. 157.
2. Shingles, p. 156.

Irritation

Two main causes, both of which are usually chronic with acute exacerbations:

1. Blepharitis – crusted or matted eyelashes, often with injected lid margins and chronic itch.
2. Allergy – usually in atopic patients with eczema.

Blepharitis

Features

This is extremely common and leads to chronic bilateral lid and ocular irritation, rather than pain, with acute exacerbations. The lashes frequently have skin debris attached to them or may be matted together.

Management

1. Advise the patient that the condition is chronic, and treatment is to relieve symptoms, but will not cure the underlying problem.
2. Stain the cornea with fluorescein, and observe under a blue light for a marginal ulcer (p. 27). There is usually localized conjunctival injection if an ulcer is present.
3. If the lids are very injected, start on chloramphenicol ointment 1% t.d.s. The patient should firmly rub this into the eyelid margins, at the base of their eyelashes for 3 weeks. There is no need to instil this into the eye.
4. Lid hygiene. Advise the patient to clean the lid margins thoroughly morning and night by pulling the skin of the outer lid margins laterally to put the lid margin under tension. With a clean lint cloth or flannel dampened with a mild solution of saline (one teaspoon of salt in a tumbler of cooled boiled water) or baby shampoo, firmly rub the margins to remove grease and debris associated with the condition. This treatment should be continued indefinitely.

Referral and follow-up

Not required in the absence of corneal pathology. If corneal staining is present, refer to the ophthalmologist within 24 hours.

Allergy

Features

This may occur acutely as a result of exposure to dust,

fur or pollen in atopic individuals, in addition to antibiotic eye drops, make-up or contact lens solution. The lids may be simply oedematous with no erythema, or there may be an associated intense skin inflammation. Not uncommon in children who have rubbed their eyes, particularly if atopic.

Management

1. If there is erythema or inflammation of the lids or periorbital tissues, treat as periorbital cellulitis (p. 150).
2. If the lids or periorbital tissues are simply swollen but not injected, this is typical of an acute allergic response, particularly if the conjunctiva is similarly swollen and appears as a pale yellow coloured bag of fluid surrounding the cornea. This usually settles spontaneously within 24 hours. If severe, oral antihistamines may speed recovery.
3. Identify any possible allergen from the history (usually grass, pollen, debris from sand pits in children).
4. Stop any antibiotic eye drops, and do not substitute another.
5. If the patient is a contact lens wearer, these should be removed, and left out until reviewed as below.
6. Advise the patient to stop using make-up, or change to a hypoallergenic variety.
7. Cold compresses are useful. Advise the patient, or parents of affected child to soak a clean flannel in cold water and place over the closed eyes.
8. Do not treat with eye drops, as these may exacerbate the problem.

Referral

Children should be discussed with the ophthalmologist immediately. If due to contact lens wear or antibiotic drops, refer to the ophthalmologist within 24 hours. All other cases may be discharged.

Follow-up

This is required only in cases that have not settled within 24 hours, and these should be referred immediately to the ophthalmologist.

Infection

1. Localized – e.g. stye, blepharitis (see below).
2. Diffuse – e.g. preseptal or orbital cellulitis (Plate 1, and p. 150).

Localized infection

Features

Stye – this is centred around an eyelash follicle and may have a pointing 'head' visible (Fig. 8.1c, p. 152).
Infected chalazion – A tender lump further away from the lid margin within the eyelid. A previously long-standing painless lump (chalazion) may have been present prior to infection (Fig. 8.1a, p. 152).
Blepharitis – see p. 146.
Dacryocystitis – infected lacrimal sac (Fig. 8.1, p. 153 and p. 163).

Management

1. Document the visual acuity in each eye.
2. If a stye, pull out the eyelashes involved. This may help to drain the abscess. Discharge on chloramphenicol 0.5% drops, q.d.s. for 10 days. If the problem is recurrent, check urine for diabetes and treat appropriately.
3. If an infected chalazion or dacryocystitis (infected lacrimal sac) is present, start on systemic antibiotics, e.g. Magnapen 500 mg q.d.s. p.o., in addition to chloramphenicol 0.5% drops q.d.s. for 10 days.

Referral and follow-up

Dacryocystitis (infected lacrimal sac) – treat as above (3), refer to ophthalmologist within 24 hours.
Styes, chalazia, blepharitis – no referral is required unless infection fails to resolve or worsens. Warn parents of affected children to return immediately if there are signs of spread or systemic illness. If a residual cyst remains following resolution of an infected chalazion, only refer routinely to the ophthalmology outpatient department if the patient wishes surgery, otherwise discharge.

Diffuse infection – orbital cellulitis

Features

Diffuse erythema and infection may follow localized infection quite rapidly, and lead to preseptal (superficial tissues) or orbital (deep tissues) cellulitis (Plate 1). The latter has a high mortality if not treated promptly.

Relevant questions

1. *Has there been any trauma?*
   Scratches and plucked eyebrows can be the original sites of infection.
2. *Is there a history of styes, previous lid infections, sinusitis or upper respiratory tract infection?*
   Orbital tissue may become involved from adjacent infected regions, particularly from the ethmoids in children.
3. *Is there malaise?*
   Particularly important in children, who can rapidly develop systemic symptoms.

Examination

1. Document visual acuity in each eye.
2. Look for source of infection, e.g. stye, scratch or plucked eyebrows.
3. Look for restriction of eye movements and ask about double vision (Fig. 3.2, p. 37). If either are present, consider orbital cellulitis. Check eye movements using a target at least 60 cm from the patient – if you get too close, you may induce physiological double vision. Painful restricted movement occurs in orbital cellulitis, and the eye itself is usually red.
4. Ensure pupil reactions are normal and that there is no afferent defect (p. 3) as a result of optic nerve compression associated with orbital cellulitis.
5. Sinus X-rays if there is a history of sinusitis.

Management and referral

1. *Children* – admit immediately for systemic antibiotics, preferably under the paediatricians. Give i.v.

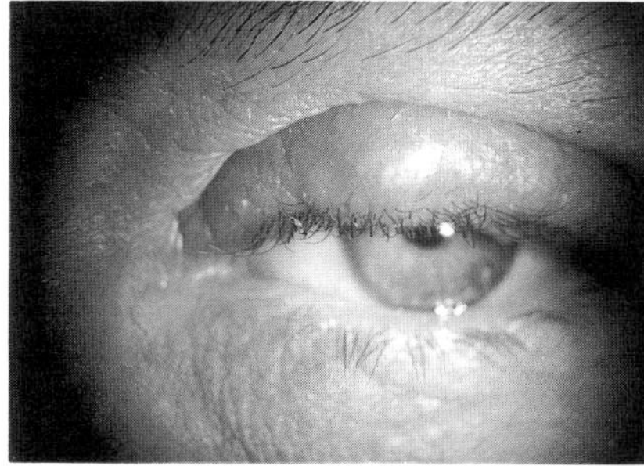

a.
Chalazion within the upper eyelid
p. 154

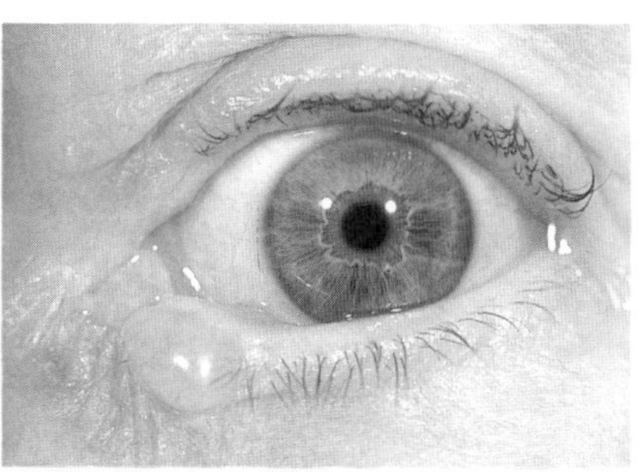

b.
Cyst of moll
p. 154

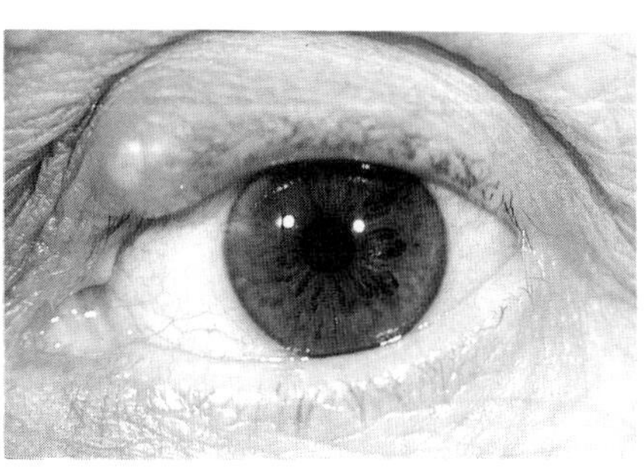

c.
Stye. p. 149
Note the presence of a 'head'

Fig. 8.1. Common lid lesions.

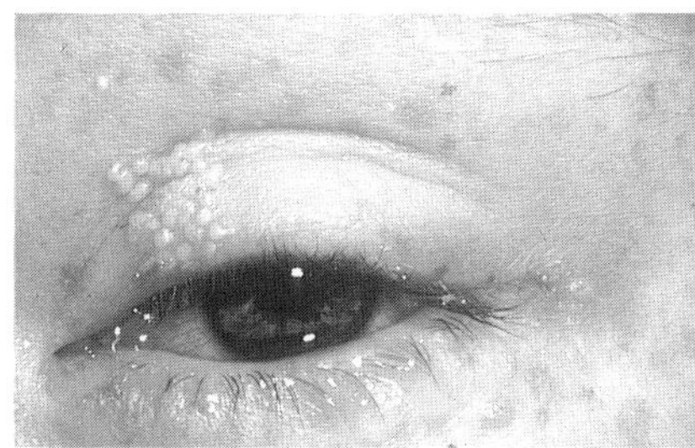

d.
Herpes simplex vesicles (examine cornea for associated dendritic ulceration, p. 27)

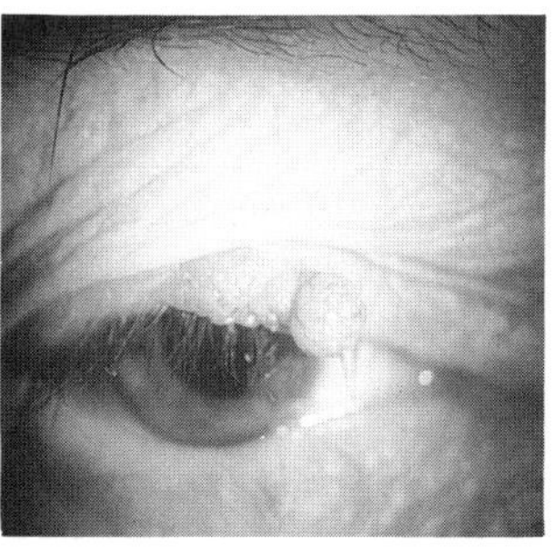

e.
Upper eyelid papilloma, p. 154

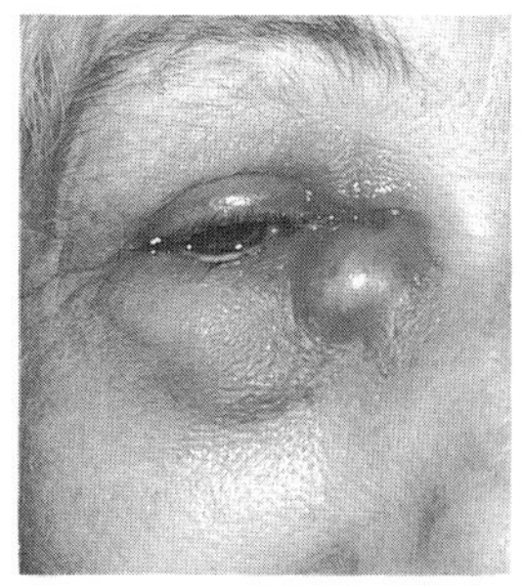

f.
Dacryocystitis infection of the lacrimal sac, p. 150 and 163. (consider lacrimal tumour)

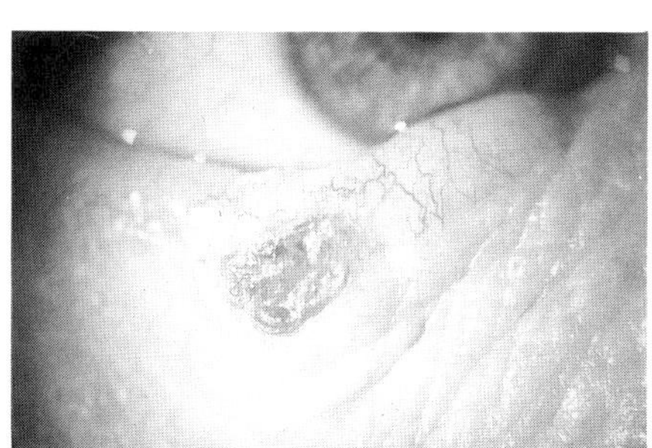

g.
Basal cell carcinoma with surface crusting p. 154

systemic antibiotics after seeking advice from paediatric physicians if a delay is likely before the child reaches the ward. Orbital computed tomography (CT) or magnetic resonance imaging (MRI) may be required.

2. *Diplopia, decreased vision or afferent pupil defect* – if any abnormal ocular findings are present, admit immediately under ophthalmologists, children are best admitted under paediatricians, for i.v. antibiotics and orbital CT or MRI.
3. *No systemic or ocular features other than lid involvement* – in an adult, treat with oral antibiotics, e.g. Magnapen 500 mg q.d.s. p.o., and refer to the ophthalmologist within 24 hours.
4. *X-ray orbit* if there is a history of sinusitis or previous trauma.

Cysts and other lumps

These are common and may have been present for months (Fig. 8.1, pp. 152–3).

Features

1. *Chalazion* – non-tender lump felt in the upper or lower eyelid. Often recurrent.
2. *Wart or papilloma* – often at the lid margin. May be flat or pedunculated. Craggy surface.
3. *Cyst of Moll* – small, clear cyst on lid margin.
4. *Basal cell carcinoma* – pearly edged ‘ulcer’ usually on lower lid. May bleed and crust over.

All of the above have usually been present for months.

Management and referral

1. *Chalazia* need only be referred to the ophthalmology outpatient department if unsightly, or if the patient complains of irritation, particularly if a contact lens wearer. If small and causing no bother, reassure (spontaneous resolution may occur) and discharge. If infected, see p. 149.
2. *Papillomata* not involving the eyelashes can be removed with cautery under local anaesthetic or simply be referred routinely to the ophthalmology outpatient department. Do not attempt surgery on children or young adults. If the patient is undecided about surgery, discharge.
3. *Cysts* can be drained by slicing with an orange needle mounted on a 2 ml syringe to act as a handle. Local anaesthetic is not required. Do not attempt this near the inferior canaliculus (medial end of lower lid). Referral is unnecessary but recurrence is common.
4. *Basal cell carcinomas* should be referred to the ophthalmology outpatient department (soon).
5. *Melanoma*. If suspected, refer to the ophthalmologist within 48 hours.
6. *Lacrimal gland enlargement* may appear as a fullness in the upper eyelid temporally, and can be palpated through the skin beneath the globe and the superior orbital rim. Refer to the ophthalmology outpatient department (soon), or discuss with the ophthalmologist if painful.
7. *Other lesions* of which you are unsure – refer routinely to the ophthalmologist. If the history suggests malignancy, e.g. growth or bleeding, arrange ophthalmology review within 48 hours.

Shingles

Features

Skin vesicles and subsequent crusting in herpes zoster ophthalmicus (HZO) may be very severe with scarring, or may present as merely a few skin vesicles. Ocular involvement does not always occur.

Management

If the underlying eye is red, or vision is reduced – see Red eye, shingles, p. 33.

Normal underlying eye

1. Treat skin with emollient cream (E45) to prevent crusting.
2. Start 'shingles pack'. Acyclovir (Zovirax) 800 mg p.o. five times daily for 1 week, if less than 2 weeks from onset.
3. Analgesia. Orally or i.m. The pain may be excruciating.
4. Neuralgia is common following shingles. The following may be effective if simple analgesia fails:
   (a) Transcutaneous nerve stimulation (TENS) – see Referral, below.
   (b) Amitriptyline – 25 mg o.d. p.o. starting dose (beware urinary retention, cardiotoxic).
   (c) Carbamazepine (Tegretol) 100 mg nocte p.o. (narrow therapeutic range).

Referral

Severe debility – admit under physicians/infectious diseases unit for support.

Normal-looking eye with lid involvement – ophthalmologist within 24 hours.
Neuralgia – Physiotherapy outpatient department for TENS. If persistent and severe, refer to neurologist (outpatient department, soon) or pain clinic if one is available. Obtain advice from physicians prior to starting amitriptyline or carbamazepine.
Red eye – see p. 33.

Entropion and ectropion

Entropion and ingrowing lashes (trichiasis)

Features

Entropion – lid has turned in on itself, allowing eyelashes to touch the eye (see Fig. 2.1a, p. 22).
Trichiasis – ingrowing, aberrent eyelashes. Can occur without entropion.

Management

1. Trichiasis only – epilate (pull out) the offending lashes with forceps.
2. If entropion is present, use steristrips to pull the lower lid off the globe (see Fig. 2.1b, p. 22). To to this:
   (a) Dry the skin.
   (b) Place one end of a steristrip on the skin just below the lashes.
   (c) Pull down gently until lashes are pulled off the globe.
   (d) Stick other end on to cheek.
   (e) Use three steristrips in a row.

3. Stain the cornea with dilute fluorescein and look for lash-induced abrasions.
4. If corneal staining is present, instil chloramphenicol ointment 1%.
5. Discharge on chloramphenicol ointment 1% t.i.d. for 5 days.

Referral

If entropion is present, refer for an ophthalmology outpatient assessment soon. If there is no entropion, but the problem is one of recurrent ingrowing lashes, organize a routine ophthalmology outpatient appointment.

Follow-up

Ophthalmologist for entropion. General practitioner for routine epilation of lashes.

Ectropion

Features

Lower lid turned out, with inner surface exposed (see Fig. 7.1, p. 142) Watering eye. Usually secondary to lax tissues in elderly individuals.

Management

1. Stain the cornea with fluorescein and look for diffuse, fine staining indicating exposure.
2. Lacri-Lube ointment t.d.s.

Referral

Corneal staining present – ophthalmology outpatients within 2 weeks.
Corneal staining absent – routine ophthalmology outpatient appointment.

Follow-up

Ophthalmologist only.

9

Tumours and tumour-like lesions

External ocular tumours

Lids – these are described under Lids on p. 154. See Fig. 8.1, p. 152.

Conjunctiva

Two main categories:

1. Pigmented lesions.
2. Red, painful or irritable lesions.

Pigmented lesions

Features

May be simple naevi or malignant melanoma. Growth, bleeding, elevated lesion or change in colour indicates potential malignancy. Benign naevi may enlarge at puberty or during pregnancy.

Management

There is no management appropriate to casualty or GP.

Referral and follow-up

1. If the lesion is new or there is evidence of malignancy, refer to ophthalmologist within 48 hours.
2. If the lesion is old with no evidence of malignancy, reassure, but advise to reattend immediately should any change occur.
3. If the patient is unsure of the duration of the lesion, refer to ophthalmology outpatient department soon, where follow-up will be arranged if required.

Red, painful or irritable lesions

Features

When near the corneal margin (limbus), these are often foci of inflammation rather than tumours, e.g. pinguecula. Nodular episcleritis (p. 31) may present as a red oedematous lump near the limbus, usually at 3 or 9 o'clock. A triangular extension of conjunctiva pointing towards the centre of the cornea is a pterygium, and is common in those who live or work in a hot, dry environment.

Management, referral and follow-up

1. Stain with fluorescein to ensure that the lesion is not due to:
   (a) A foreign body (p. 18)
   (b) Abrasion (p. 16)
   (c) Ulcer (p. 27).
2. If painful, and not due to a foreign body, abrasion or ulcer, refer to the ophthalmologist within 24

hours. If very painful (possible scleritis), discuss immediately.
3. Consider episcleritis. Treat as described on p. 31.

Periorbital and orbital

1. Proptosis
2. Red abscess next to nose (dacryocystitis)
3. Non-tender, non-inflamed mass next to nose (mucocoele)

Proptosis

Features

Dysthyroid disease is the most common cause (p. 47). The eye may be red with conjunctival chemosis (waterlogging). Restriction of eye movements is common, and diplopia (double vision) may occur. Consider orbital mass such as tumour or abscess.

Management, referral and follow-up

For examination, see under Thyroid, on p. 47.

1. Painless proptosis with normal visual acuity and pupils should be referred to the ophthalmologist within 24 hours.
2. All others should be discussed with and admitted under the ophthalmologists immediately.

Red 'abscess' next to nose (dacryocystitis)

Features

Situated just below the inner canthus (nasal side of the eyelids), this is usually dacryocystitis, an infection of the lacrimal sac (Fig. 8.1f, p. 153). There is frequently a long history of watering eye with recurrent infections.

Management, referral and follow-up

1. Magnapen 500 mg q.d.s. p.o. and refer to the ophthalmologist within 24 hours.
2. Do not lance (leave this to the ophthalmologist) as this may cause a fistula and detrimentally affect final outcome.

Non-inflamed, non-tender fluctuant mass next to nose (mucocoele)

Features

This is usually a mucocoele within the lacrimal sac and is associated with an ipsilateral watering eye. If gentle pressure is applied, mucopus frequently exits from the cannaliculi.

Management, referral and follow-up

Refer to ophthalmology outpatient department within a few weeks. No immediate management required.

Internal ocular tumour – iris

Pigmented lesions

Features

If small and multiple, these are usually iris freckles and are long-standing.

If single, larger than about 1 mm, and particularly if causing distortion of the round pupil, consider melanoma.

Management, referral and follow-up

1. Long-standing iris freckles require no intervention. Reassure and discharge.
2. If any increase in number or size of freckles, or any suspicion of malignancy, refer to ophthalmology outpatient department within a week (melanomas of the iris do not invariably require excision).

Non-pigmented lesions

Features

Iris cysts are rare, may look solid and can occur months or years after surgery or trauma.

Amelanotic melanomas are very rare.

Management, referral and follow-up

Refer routinely to the ophthalmology outpatient department. If there is any suspicion of malignancy (growth, change in colour, pupil distortion), refer to the ophthalmologist within a week.

Retina and choroid

Features – adult

Presentation is usually as a result of decreased vision or 'shadowing' in the visual field and rarely due to secondary glaucoma or haemorrhage within the eye.

1. *Melanoma* – this is the most common primary internal ocular tumour in adults, and arises from the choroid. It usually appears as a dark elevated fixed mass which may be quite anterior in the eye (ciliary body tumour) or further back. Localized large 'conjunctival' blood vessels (feeder vessels) often indicate an anterior underlying tumour. A retinal detachment may overlie the tumour.
2. *Secondaries (metastases)* – the most common internal ocular tumour overall. Rapid growth is common. Usually at the posterior pole (optic disc and macula), often pale elevated lesions with poorly defined edges. Primary is usually breast in females, bronchus in males. Field defects may be present due to cerebral metastases.

Features – child

Retinoblastoma is the most common primary intraocular tumour in children, but nevertheless is very rare. A white pupil reflex (leukocoria) or squint is usually the reason for presentation.

Management, referral and follow-up

1. Refer all cases to the ophthalmologist within 48 hours.
2. If retinoblastoma is suspected (children), all siblings and both parents should also be examined by the ophthalmologist.
3. If secondaries are suspected (adult), refer to relevant specialty for investigation of possible primary.
4. Chest X-ray for melanomas and secondaries (adults).
5. GP or casualty follow-up is not required.

10 Postoperative problems

Problems may occur in the immediate postoperative period or months later (Fig. 10.1, p. 165).

Pain or acutely reduced vision should be discussed immediately with the ophthalmologist.

Relevant questions

1. *When did the patient have the operation?*
   The problem may be long-standing or unrelated to previous surgery.
2. *What type of operation was it?*
   Was it intraocular (cataract extraction, trabeculectomy for glaucoma, some retinal detachment repairs, corneal graft) or extraocular (squint repair, lid surgery)?
3. *Is the eye painful or just irritable?*
   Although pain is quite common following retinal detachment surgery and cryotherapy, it is uncommon following most other eye operations. If following intraocular surgery, this may indicate intraocular infection (endophthalmitis). Irritation is usually caused by sutures (Fig. 10.1a), and may occur months or years after the operation.
4. *Is vision reduced?*
   An acute reduction in visual acuity following intraocular surgery may indicate endophthalmitis, particularly if associated with pain. A gradual reduction over months is not uncommon following

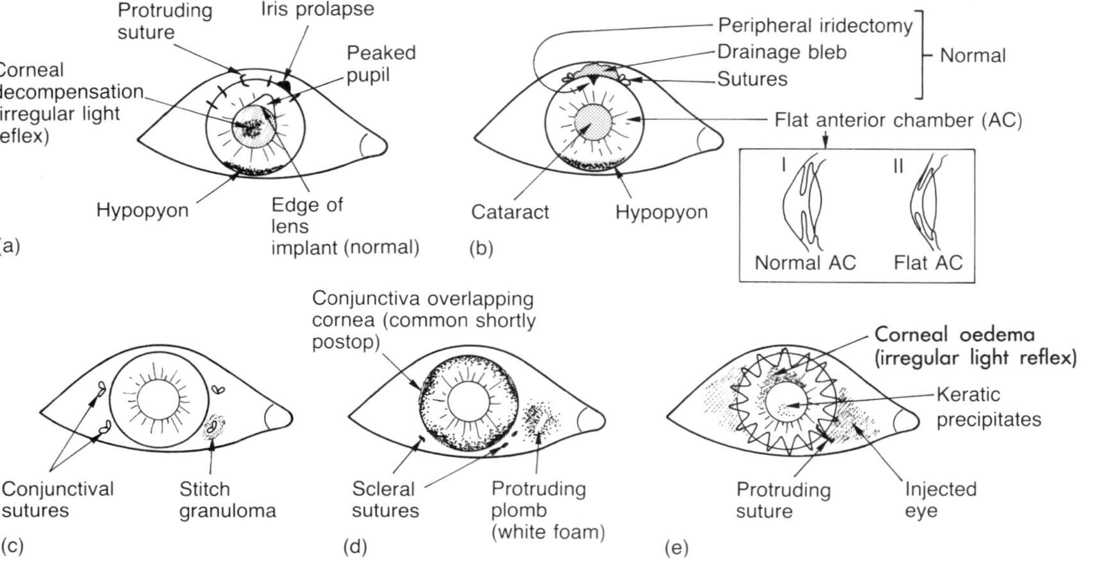

Fig. 10.1. Postoperative appearances and complications. (a) cataract; (b) trabeculectomy; (c) squint; (d) retinal detachment; (e) corneal graft.

cataract extraction, and is usually due to membrane thickening behind the lens implant.

5. *Is the patient on any treatment to the operated eye?* Patients may omit treatment postoperatively. Refer to Chapter 11, p. 178.

Examination

External

Lid oedema and erythema are common after retinal detachment surgery or cryotherapy (freezing applied to the globe or lids) for up to a week post operatively, but there should be no discharge. Orbital cellulitis may occur but is rare (Plate 1 and p. 150).

The eye itself is frequently injected (red) for 2–3 weeks following most surgery although modern cataract surgery now leads to little post-operative inflammation.

Visual acuity

Very variable. Document using a pinhole (p. 2). A history of reduced vision *since* surgery is more important than just poor vision. If there is associated pain, consider endophthalmitis (internal ocular infection).

Pupil

Often pharmacologically dilated. Ask to see the patient's eye drops if he or she has them (if not, refer to p. 178). Look at the red reflex (look through an ophthalmoscope at the pupil from about 60 cm – you should see a red reflex through the pupil. Absence of this reflex in association with pain and reduced vision is associated with intraocular infection (endophthalmitis).

Cornea and sclera

The cornea should be clear. Corneal haze may indicate raised intraocular pressure or graft rejection. A layer of white cells may be seen obscuring the inferior iris. This is a hypopyon (pus in the eye, Plate 9) and indicates intraocular infection, which may occur any time following an operation, but is most common within a few days of intraocular surgery – usually a cataract extraction. A cyst (drainage bleb) at the upper corneoscleral junction is normal after glaucoma surgery (Fig. 10.1b, p. 168). If the cyst is red and tender, consider infection. Dark tissue protruding through the superior corneoscleral junction following cataract surgery indicates prolapse of the iris (Fig. 10.1a, p. 168).

Cataract surgery

Features (Fig. 10.1a, p. 168)

Serious signs and symptoms

These usually occur within the first week, but can occur later.

1. Pain (as opposed to irritation).
2. Sudden reduction of visual acuity since the operation.
3. Loss of red reflex.
4. Hazy cornea.

5. Hypopyon.
6. Iris tissue visible in wound line (iris prolapse).

Less serious signs and symptoms

These may occur immediately or several months postoperatively.

- Irritation – or gritty sensation – often due to sutures. These may be visible after staining with fluorescein at the upper junction between the cornea and sclera, just under the upper lid. Do not attempt to remove these.
- Gradual loss of vision – this is usually due to membrane formation behind the lens implant, but be aware of retinal detachment (p. 79).

Management

No management is appropriate in a GP or casualty setting. All cases should be referred as below.

Referral

Serious signs and symptoms – immediately to the ophthalmologist.
Less serious signs and symptoms – refer to ophthalmology outpatient department (soon). If retinal detachment is suspected, see p. 79.

Follow-up

Will be undertaken by the ophthalmologist.

Pitfall

Failure to recognize and urgently refer endophthalmitis (decreased vision, red eye, pain).

Glaucoma surgery (trabeculectomy)

Features (Fig. 10.1b, p. 168)

Signs and symptoms are as for cataract surgery above. A cystic swelling at the upper corneoscleral junction is a normal finding (bleb).

Management and referral

As for cataract above.
Look at the bleb site. If this is red or tender, infection may be present. Discuss immediately with the ophthalmologist.

Follow-up

Ophthalmologist will arrange this.

Pitfall

As for cataract above.

Squint surgery

Features (Fig. 10.1c, p. 168)

Pain and discomfort are common for up to a week. The lids may be oedematous. Conjunctival sutures may be visible to each side of the cornea horizontally. Do not attempt to remove these. It is not uncommon for a residual squint to remain following surgery.

Management

1. *Purulent discharge present* – start on chloramphenicol 0.5% or gentamicin 0.3% drops 2-hourly.
2. *No discharge* – reassure patient that discomfort will settle over a few days.

Referral

Children – ophthalmology opinion within 12 hours.
Purulent discharge present – treat as above, review by ophthalmologists within 24 hours.
No discharge – reassure and advise to reattend only if symptoms worsen.

Retinal detachment surgery

Features (Fig. 10.1d, p. 168)

Pain, discomfort and lid swelling are not uncommon for up to a week following surgery. Double vision may occur. Reduced vision may be due to inflammation or re-detachment. An adequate fundal view is often difficult.

Management

Referral only. No active management is appropriate for the GP or casualty officer.

Referral

Any patient complaining of new signs or symptoms following detachment surgery should be discussed with and seen by the ophthalmologist within 24 hours.

Corneal graft surgery

Features (Fig. 10.1e, p. 168)

The cornea may look creased for several weeks postoperatively, and vision is frequently markedly reduced. Pain, further reduction in vision *since* operation, or redness may signal graft rejection.

Management and referral

Pain, reduced vision, red eye – discuss immediately with ophthalmologist. No active management is appropriate for the GP or casualty officer.

Lid surgery

The most common lid operations are:

1. Cyst removal – usually a chalazion (this is in fact a granuloma).
2. Entropion (lid turning in) or ectropion (lid turning out) repair.
3. Ptosis repair.

Problems usually relate to infection, recurrence of the original problem or wound dehiscence.

Lid infection – children

Features

Localized infection may rapidly spread into a preseptal cellulitis (p. 150).

Management

1. Localized infection – chloramphenicol drops 0.5% 2-hourly for 2 days then q.d.s. for 1 week.
2. Diffuse infection – discuss immediately with the ophthalmologist as these cases frequently require admission and intravenous antibiotics (p. 150). Older children – treat as adult.

Referral

To the ophthalmologist immediately in diffuse infection. Localized infection should be seen by the ophthalmologist if not obviously settling within 24–48 hours.

Follow-up

Localized infection – review the following day.

Lid infection – adults

Features

As for children.

Management

1. Localized infection – chloramphenicol 0.5% drops 2-hourly for 2 days then q.d.s for 1 week.
2. Diffuse infection – if erythema or swelling extends beyond a small localized area, treat with systemic antibiotics, e.g. Magnapen 500 mg q.d.s. p.o. in addition to topical antibiotics, as above.

Referral

Localized infection – not required if settling within 24–48 hours.
Diffuse infection – ophthalmology outpatient department within 24 hours.

Follow-up

Review within 24 hours to ensure adequate response to antibiotics.

Recurrence of cysts, entropion, ectropion

Cysts – if small and cosmetically acceptable, reassure and discharge, otherwise refer to the ophthalmology outpatient department routinely.

Entropion – if lashes are touching the corneal surface, tape down the bottom lid. To do this, pull down the skin just below the lid until the lashes are pulled away from the cornea. Use steristrips or tape to hold it in this position (Fig. 2.1, p. 22). Prescribe chloramphenicol 1% b.d. ointment and refer to the ophthalmologist within 48 hours.
Ectropion – stain the cornea with dilute fluorescein. If fine diffuse staining is present, usually on the lower third of the corneal surface, treat with Lacri-Lube ointment t.d.s. Refer to the ophthalmology outpatient department (soon if corneal staining present, routine otherwise).

Wound dehiscence

Stain the cornea with fluorescein. Treat diffuse staining with chloramphenicol ointment 1% t.d.s.

A corneal abrasion may be present if sutures are in contact with the corneal surface, in which case treat simply as an abrasion (p. 16). Refer all cases to the ophthalmologist within 24 hours for further repair.

11
Eye drops and drugs

Patients frequently present with eye problems which are already being treated, but fail to bring their medications and have no knowledge of the treatment they are on.

This chapter incorporates:

1. List of commonly used eye drops
2. Common postoperative drop regimes
3. Brief information on use of individual drops

Common eye drops and drugs

The following drops (*g*), ointments (*oc*) and drugs are frequently used:

Antibiotics

g Chloramphenicol 0.5% – 'yellow-top bottle'
oc Chloromycetin (chloramphenicol 1%) – mauve tube
g Genticin, oc Genticin 0.3% (both gentamicin 0.3%)
oc Fucithalmic (fusidic acid 1%)
oc Aureomycin (chlortetracycline hydrochloride 1%)

Antivirals

oc Zovirax (acyclovir 3%) – 'blue tube'

Steroids

g *Maxidex* (dexamethasone 0.1%)
g *Betnesol* (betamethasone 0.1%; Betnesol-N includes neomycin 0.5%)
g *Pred Forte* (prednisolone acetate 1%) – white ('milky drop') solution
g *Predsol* (prednisolone sodium phosphate 0.5%)
g *FML* (fluoromethalone 0.1%; infrequently used)

Hayfever-related

g *Opticrom* (sodium cromoglycate 2%)
g *Alomide* (lodoxamide 0.1%)

Glaucoma

g *Timoptol* (timolol maleate 0.25–0.5%)
g *Betagan* (levobunolol hydrochloride 0.5% + polyvinyl alcohol (Liquifilm) 1.4%)
g *Betoptic* (betaxolol 0.5%)
g *Pilocarpine* (pilocarpine hydrochloride 0.5–4.0%)
g *Propine* (dipivefrine hydrochloride 0.1%)
g *Ganda* (guanethidine 1–3% + adrenaline 0.2–0.5%; rare now)
Diamox Diamox SR (acetazolamide 250 mg) tablet or orange capsule.
Diamox – parenteral (acetazolamide 500 mg vial) i.v.

Pupil dilators (mydriatics and cycloplegics)

g *Mydrilate* (cyclopentolate hydrochloride 0.5%)
g *Minims Cyclopentolate* (cyclopentolate hydrochloride 0.5–1.0%)
g *Minims Tropicamide* (tropicamide 0.5–1.0%)

gAtropine, oc Atropine (both atropine 1%) – 'red-top bottle'
g Homatropine (homatropine hydrobromide 1%; infrequently used)

Lubricants

g Hypromellose (hypromellose 0.3%)
g Tears Naturale (dextran 70 0.1% + hypromellose 0.3%)
g Artificial Tears (hydroxyethylcellulose 0.44%)
g Liquifilm (polyvinyl alcohol 1.4%)
oc Lacri-Lube (white soft and liquid paraffin)
oc Ilube (acetylcysteine 5% + hypromellose 0.35%; infrequently used)

Anaesthetics

g Benoxinate (oxybuprocaine hydrochloride 0.4%)
g Amethocaine (amethocaine hydrochloride 0.5%)

Eye stains

g Fluorescein (fluorescein sodium 1–2%)

Common postoperative regimes

Regimes vary. The following are common.

Cataract surgery

g Maxidex, Betnesol or Pred Forte q.d.s. for 2 weeks, thereafter b.d. for 4 weeks then stop.

g Chloramphenicol 0.5% q.d.s. for 2 weeks, thereafter b.d. for 4 weeks then stop.
g Mydrilate t.d.s. for 2 weeks then stop (frequently not used at all).

Glaucoma patients should continue to use their glaucoma drops following cataract surgery (exception pilocarpine; discuss with ophthalmologist).

Glaucoma surgery (trabeculectomy)

g Maxidex, Betnesol or Pred Forte q.d.s. for 2 weeks, thereafter b.d. for 4 weeks then stop.
g Chloramphenicol 0.5% q.d.s. for 2 weeks, thereafter b.d. for 4 weeks then stop.
g Mydrilate t.d.s. for 3 weeks then stop or g Atropine 1% b.d. for 2 weeks, then stop.

Glaucoma drops are usually stopped to the operated eye immediately following surgery, but must be continued in the unoperated eye if previously used.

Squint surgery

oc Chloramphenicol 1% t.d.s. for 2 weeks then stop.
Occasionally g Predsol and g chloramphenicol 0.5% both q.d.s. for 2 weeks then stop.
Often no medication postoperatively.

Retinal detachment surgery

g Maxidex, Betnesol or Pred Forte q.d.s. 2 weeks, thereafter b.d. for 4 weeks then stop.

g Chloramphenicol 0.5% q.d.s. for 2 weeks, thereafter b.d. for 4 weeks then stop.
Atropine 1% b.d. for 2 weeks, then stop.
Oral analgesia.

Dacryocystorhinostomy (for watering eyes)

Often no therapy required postoperatively. The following however may be used:

g Chloramphenicol q.d.s. for 2 weeks, then stop.
Magnapen 500 mg q.d.s. p.o. for 10 days.

Brief notes on each common drug

Antibiotics

Chloramphenicol

Bacteriostatic only. Occasional allergic response. Frequency q.d.s. but can increase to hourly. First-line treatment in simple conjunctivitis.

Genticin

Bacteriocidal. More frequent allergies. If chloramphenicol fails, take swabs (bacterial) then use q.d.s. or hourly in severe infections.

Fucithalmic

Broad-spectrum. Only requires b.d. application. First-line treatment in simple conjunctivitis.

Aureomycin

Use in suspected chlamydial disease – q.d.s. for 3 weeks. Treat partner.

Antivirals

Zovirax

Frequency five times daily for 5 days. Low corneal toxicity compared with other antivirals. Do not use skin preparation Zovirax in the eye.

Steroids

Maxidex

Potent steroid and widely used. Frequency from hourly in severe inflammation to once daily. Usually q.d.s. postoperatively. May cause raised intraocular pressure.

Betnesol

Less potent than Maxidex. Usually q.d.s. May cause raised intraocular pressure.

Pred Forte

Potent steroid with high penetration into anterior chamber. Usually q.d.s. but may be used hourly in severe inflammation. May cause raised intraocular pressure.

Predsol

Less potent than the above. Very weak concentrations may be used long-term in corneal scarring due to old viral keratitis. May cause raised intraocular pressure. Frequency from q.d.s. to o.d.

FML

Infrequently used. Causes less intraocular pressure rise than other steroids.

Hayfever-related

Opticrom

Can take up to 3 weeks before taking effect. Usual frequency q.d.s. Long-term use, but may be restricted to hayfever season.

Alomide

Fast onset of action. Usual frequency q.d.s.

Glaucoma

Patients should not stop antiglaucoma treatment unless instructed to do so by an ophthalmologist (unless breathlessness occurs with β-blockers, e.g. Timoptol).

Timoptol

Contraindicated in chronic obstructive airways disease and heart block. Frequency b.d.

Betagan

As for Timoptol.

Betopic

As for Timoptol.

Pilocarpine

Causes pupil miosis (small pupil). Headaches and poor vision in the dark are initially common. Infrequent allergic reaction (local effect). Frequency q.d.s.

Propine

Causes pupil dilatation (enlarged pupil). Allergic conjunctivitis not uncommon. Frequency b.d.

Ganda

Rarely used. Higher strengths may cause conjunctival fibrosis.

Diamox

i.v. – 500 mg powder dissolved in 10 ml water for injections. For rapid intraocular pressure reduction. p.o. – 250–500 mg tablets. Usual maximum 1 g/day. Slow-release preparation available, frequency o.d. or b.d.

Pupil dilators (and ciliary muscle relaxants)

Mydrilate

Duration up to 12 hours. Will cause blurring, particularly for reading. Advise against driving after instillation. Beware in the elderly – particularly if long-sighted (check glasses – act as magnifying lenses) as you may precipitate angle-closure glaucoma (rare in practice, however). Usual frequency b.d. or t.d.s.

Atropine

Duration up to 2 weeks. Allergy may occur. Used in children to measure for spectacles. Beware of systemic effects – tachycardia, flushing, dry mouth and delirium. Lethal doses in young children may be reached using eye drops.

Homatropine

Infrequently used. As for Mydrilate – but has longer duration of action.

Lubricants

Hypromellose, Tears Naturale, Artificial Tears, Liquifilm Tears

All may be used for symptomatic relief as frequently as necessary – even half-hourly. Allergy to preservative may occur.

Lacri-Lube

Usual frequency t.d.s. in addition to drops as above in severe dry eye. Less severe cases may only require one application at night. Blurs vision transiently (ointment) and may be unsightly (oily appearance around eyes).

Ilube

Infrequently used. Discomfort if used long term. Used to dissolve excess mucus in tear film – usually with dry eyes. Frequency b.d. to t.d.s.

Anaesthetics

Benoxinate

More comfortable than amethocaine. Warn patient it will sting for 30 seconds or so. Do not give to patient to take away, particularly in corneal abrasions – it will slow down corneal healing and put the eye in greater danger of further damage.

Amethocaine

Uncomfortable for 30 seconds – warn patient. Do not give to patient – reasons as for benoxinate above. Repeated use may lead to extensive corneal and conjunctival epithelial defects which are extremely painful and slow to heal.

Stains

Fluorescein

Drop form or dried onto a strip (Fluoret). Use sparingly. If concentrated, i.e. 2% in minims dropper, it will not fluoresce under blue (cobalt) light, thus corneal defects may be missed. Dilute with a drop of saline if required, although the patient's tear film is usually a sufficient diluent.

Glossary

Anatomy

Anterior chamber	The space between the posterior surface of the cornea and the lens which is filled with aqueous fluid
Ciliary body	The circumferential muscle body at the root of the iris
Conjunctival fornices	The gutters formed by the conjunctiva as it curves back on itself between the globe and the inner layer of the eyelids
Fundus	The retina and optic disc
Lens	The crystalline lens is located just posterior to the iris. A phakic individual is one with the natural lens. Aphakia describes absence of this lens and pseudophakia indicates the presence of an artificial lens implant following cataract surgery
Limbus	The junction between clear cornea and sclera
Macula	The area of retina which is responsible for central vision, located just temporal to the optic disc

Posterior segment	The space between the back of the lens and the retina, containing vitreous
Punctum	The lacrimal punctum is a small elevated mound located at the medial end of the upper and lower lids at the lid margin

Red eye

Chemosis	Oedema of the conjunctiva
Dendritic	The branching pattern of corneal ulcers due to herpes simplex
Ectropion	Turning out of the lower lid
Endophthalmitis	Intraocular infection
Entropion	Inturning of the lower lid, leading to contact between the lashes and the cornea Upper-lid entropion may also occur
Episcleritis	Inflammation of the superficial outer vascular coat of the eye – the episclera
Hyphaema	Blood level in the anterior chamber
Hypopyon	Pus level in anterior chamber

Iritis	Inflammation of the iris
Keratoconjunctivitis	Infection of cornea (keratitis) and conjunctiva simultaneously
Subtarsal	Under the eyelid – as in subtarsal foreign body (STFB)
Uveitis	Inflammation of uveal tissue, of which the iris is the anterior portion, hence anterior uveitis is used synonymously with iritis
Trichiasis	Ingrowing eyelashes which abrade the cornea

Visual symptoms

Afferent pupil defect (APD)	Detailed description on p. 3
AION	Anterior ischaemic optic neuropathy
Amblyopia	Reduced vision in an anatomically normal eye ('lazy eye')
BRVO	Branch retinal vein occlusion
CRAO	Central retinal artery occlusion
CRVO	Central retinal vein occlusion

Homonymous hemianopia	Field loss affecting either both left or right fields, as opposed to bitemporal hemianopia, which describes loss in the temporal field of both eyes
IOP	Intraocular pressure
Myopia	Short sight
Optic chiasm	Overlying the pituitary; the site where both optic nerves meet and nasal fibres cross over
Optic neuritis	Inflammation of the optic nerve posterior to the optic disc
Proliferative	As in proliferative retinopathy – new vessel growth seen on the optic disc or retina
RD	Retinal detachment
PVD	Posterior vitreous detachment

Trauma

Blow-out fracture	Prolapse of ocular contents through orbital floor into maxillary sinus
Commotio retinae	Retinal bruising and oedema

Infraorbital nerve	Supplies sensation to ipsilateral cheek and upper teeth

Watering eye

Nasolacrimal system	Drainage system for tears, starting with the lacrimal puncta on the upper and lower lids medially, via the lacrimal sac, terminating in the nasolacrimal canal which drains into the back of the nose
Stenosis	Closure or narrowing, e.g. punctal stenosis

Lids

Chalazion	Lipogranulomatous 'cyst' within the body of the upper or lower lid

Tumours of eye

Dacryocystitis	Infection of the lacrimal sac
Mucocoele	Non-infected lacrimal sac filled with mucus

Index